the Wellness Garden

GROW, EAT, AND WALK YOUR WAY TO BETTER HEALTH

SHAWNA CORONADO

COOL
SPRINGS
PRESS

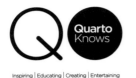

Quarto Knows

Inspiring | Educating | Creating | Entertaining

Brimming with creative inspiration, how-to projects, and useful information to enrich your everyday life, Quarto Knows is a favorite destination for those pursuing their interests and passions. Visit our site and dig deeper with our books into your area of interest: Quarto Creates, Quarto Cooks, Quarto Homes, Quarto Lives, Quarto Drives, Quarto Explores, Quarto Gifts, or Quarto Kids.

First published in 2017 by Cool Springs Press, an imprint of The Quarto Group,
401 Second Avenue North, Suite 310, Minneapolis, MN 55401 USA.
T (612) 344-8100 F (612) 344-8692 www.QuartoKnows.com

Cool Springs Press titles are also available at discount for retail, wholesale, promotional, and bulk purchase. For details, contact the Special Sales Manager by email at specialsales@quarto.com or by mail at The Quarto Group, Attn: Special Sales Manager, 401 Second Avenue North, Suite 310, Minneapolis, MN 55401 USA.

10 9 8 7 6 5 4 3 2 1

ISBN: 978-1-59186-694-7

Library of Congress Cataloging-in-Publication Data
Names: Coronado, Shawna, author.
Title: The wellness garden : grow, eat, and walk your way to better health / Shawna Coronado.
Description: Minneapolis, MN : Cool Springs Press, 2017. | Includes index.
Identifiers: LCCN 2017019288 | ISBN 9781591866947 (pb)
Subjects: LCSH: Organic gardening. | Gardening--Therapeutic use. | Health promotion.
Classification: LCC SB453.5 .C665 2017 | DDC 635/.0484--dc23
LC record available at https://lccn.loc.gov/2017019288

Printed in China

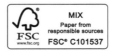

MIX
Paper from responsible sources
FSC® C101537

DISCLAIMER: The information in this book is for educational purposes only. It is not intended to replace the advice of a physician, nutritionist, or medical practitioner. Please see your health-care provider before beginning any new health program. The author and publisher specifically disclaim all responsibility for any liability, loss, or risk, personal or otherwise, which is incurred as a consequence, directly or indirectly, of the use and application of any of the contents of this book.

Acquiring Editor:
Mark Johanson

Project Manager:
Alyssa Bluhm

Art Director:
Cindy Samargia Laun

Cover Design:
Lisa Amaroso

Page Design and Layout:
Diana Boger

On the cover: Franz Peter Rudolf/Shutterstock (top); GAP Gardens/Torie Chugg (bottom)

On the back cover:
Shawna Coronado

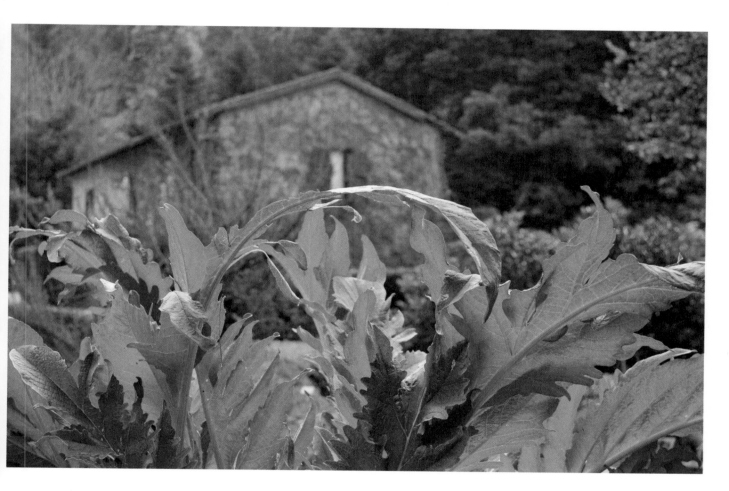

These artichoke leaves play a role in the gardens at the Orto Botanic di Roma in Rome, Italy: they are beautiful, they are organic, they are full of nutrition. Most importantly, beautiful vegetables ask the visitor to slow down, take a long look, and breathe in the outdoors while walking through the garden.

CONTENTS

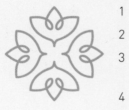

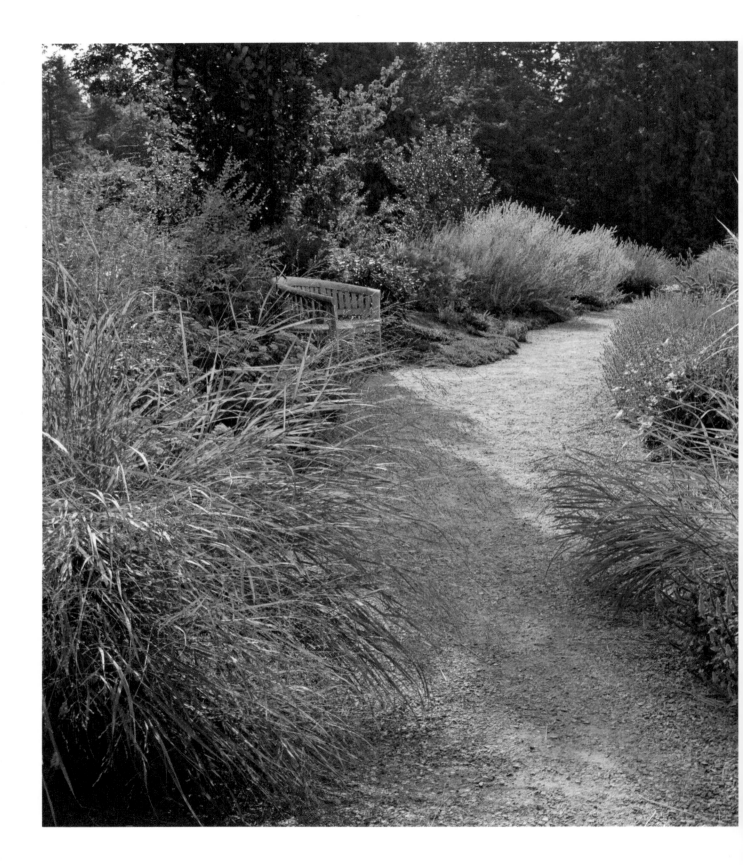

INTRODUCTION:
WHAT IS A WELLNESS GARDEN?

THERE IS NO place I feel better than when I am surrounded by plants and nature. Gardening and spending time outdoors is, at least in my mind, the single most wonderful thing a person can do to feel well. That's what this book is all about: defining and finding your own personal wellness and living mindfully with nature in order to reduce symptoms of common health conditions.

OPPOSITE: While growing your own garden is important, visiting municipal parks, green spaces, and gardens can also be a healthful experience. Public gardens offer walking paths and therapeutic landscapes. Drought-tolerant perennials such as Russian sage, nepeta, veronica, and ornamental grasses found at the Bellevue Botanical Garden in Washington State offer color, scent, and sound that usher visitors through the garden.

With the help of my nutritionist and doctors, I overcame debilitating pain from severe degenerative osteoarthritis by changing my lifestyle to incorporate better nutrition through an anti-inflammatory diet, while gardening and exercising in ways that were proactive for my condition. This wellness transition has been life-altering for me on an intimate, emotional level as well as on a physical level.

Since I have discovered a lifestyle with significantly less pain, every day feels a little better, and I enjoy and appreciate my daily existence more than I ever did in the past. This transition began with gardening, but also includes diet and exercise. Because of this positive change in my own

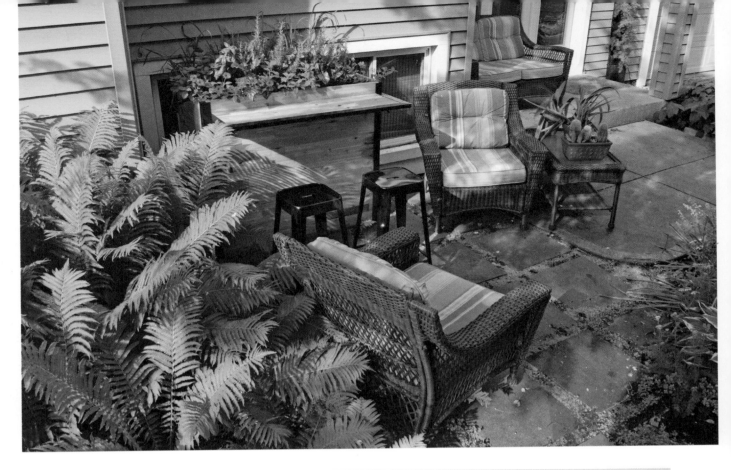

ABOVE: My front patio herbal garden bar view shows how easy it is to creatively elevate garden beds while incorporating herb and vegetable elements. This garden brings a sense of green beauty and restorative calm to a patio or seating area, exemplifying wellness.

RIGHT: A wellness garden provides a mindful experience; it offers beauty, exercise, and restoration. Harvesting nutritious foods, therapeutic scents, and pleasant sounds from that garden can add to the space's potential to heal injury and relieve anxiety. This florific summer path at the Chicago Botanic Garden ends at the Carillon Bells, which play during summer evenings.

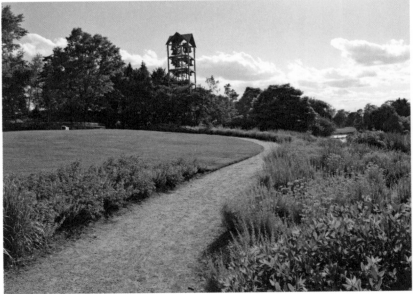

life, I want to inspire others to find similar relief, particularly with inflammation-generated chronic pain, but with other disorders as well. Reducing symptoms such as chronic pain, depression, and weight gain associated with conditions like arthritis, diabetes, high blood pressure, obesity, fibromyalgia, heart disease, and many other types of maladies without heavy medications is possible with smart diet, exercise, and lifestyle changes. I hope this book, *The Wellness Garden*, will help you explore and discover new ways to improve your lifestyle so that you can feel better every day.

Changing your lifestyle is challenging. But it is worth all the effort because a wellness lifestyle allows you to enjoy the specific dietary advantages of growing fresh herbs and vegetables in the garden, while encouraging you to spend more time exercising in the fresh air. Your gardening hobby can be translated into an experience that changes your life for the better.

My goal with this book is to inspire you to improve your overall health and fight a host of ailments that have become too common today. The good news is that living a wellness lifestyle, based on the principles discussed in this book, has worked for me. Even better: it can work for you too.

DEFINING WELLNESS

What exactly is *wellness*? According to many dictionaries, it is "the state of being in good physical and mental health." Spiritually and physically, however, wellness is a more elusive term. According to The Wellness Institute, there is a general consensus that, "Wellness is a conscious, self-directed and evolving

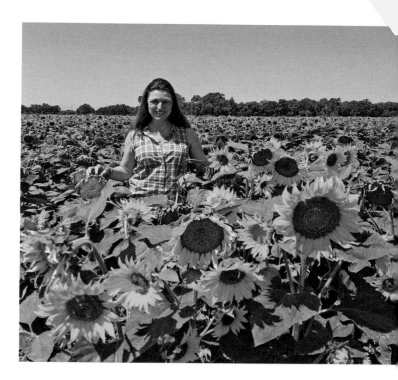

I was diagnosed with severe degenerative osteoarthritis, which led to a personal journey to rediscover wellness. In the process, I discovered that wellness is directly connected to growing my garden, regular walking and stretching exercises, as well as the specific food I consumed. These discoveries led to developing the Wellness Lifestyle, focusing my energies in the garden and on my diet, which in turn lowered my osteoarthritis pain levels and changed my quality of life.

process of achieving full potential. Wellness is multidimensional and holistic, encompassing lifestyle, mental, and spiritual well-being, and the environment; [and that] Wellness is positive and affirming. . . . *Wellness is an active process through which people become aware of, and make choices toward, a more successful existence.*"

In plain terms, the word "wellness" truly embraces an ever-changing and expanding lifestyle which involves eating healthier,

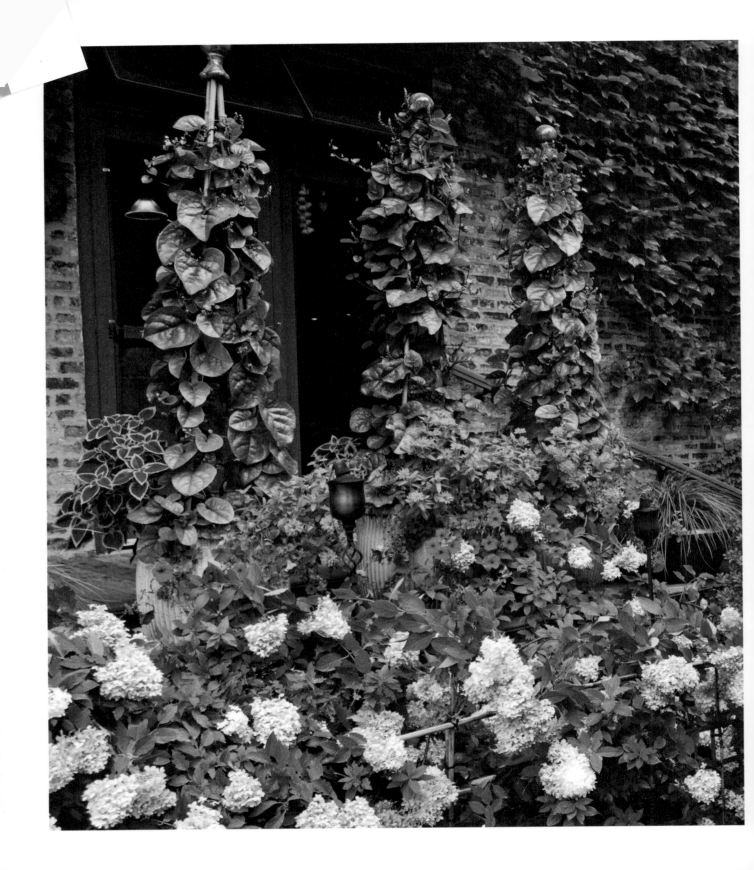

exercising regularly, and finding an emotional balance in life. It is being healthier and happier on a daily basis. Perhaps the actual process of living well is more about the journey—truly being present for our life journey—and not about the final destination in itself. Wellness is a lifestyle journey we should all practice.

FINDING MY WELLNESS

Gardening, when done wisely and with your particular physical concerns in mind, is incredibly good for your health. Benefits include being in nature, regular exercise, and growing nutritionally rich food. But gardening was also a wake-up call for me.

In my heyday as a gardener, I planted approximately 3,000 vegetables on my property every season. My crowning glory was a front lawn vegetable garden that produced 550 pounds of food per year that I donated to the local food pantry. In 2015, I dug in and planted my 3,000 vegetables. But when I was done, I discovered I could barely move. Normally, I suffered muscle soreness after planting all those vegetables, but this time I experienced debilitating pain which left me sobbing and unable to sleep. Pain medication did not help. Stretches did not help. Nothing helped. I spiraled into a depression that

OPPOSITE: An integral part of finding wellness can be through gardening. It provides physical activity, but also functions as an emotional connection to nature. Here are three Malabar spinach tower-garden containers grown on chef Rick Bayless's porch just next to his kitchen so he can pluck spinach as needed. Spinach towers are truly ornamental edible patio gardens: they function as fresh food while providing an attractive view from the kitchen.

summer and finally conceded that I needed to see a medical specialist.

THE DIAGNOSIS

At the doctor's office, I expected to be told that I had a run-of-the-mill muscle problem and would need physical therapy. Much to my surprise, the doctor asked for X-rays and confirmed a diagnosis of severe degenerative osteoarthritis of the spine, also known as degenerative joint disease. The cartilage that was supposed to be between the vertebrae of my spine had virtually disintegrated in my back and upper neck, and there is no cure. My neck is permanently malformed, and the cartilage will not grow back between the vertebrae within my back. This causes pain because bone is constantly rubbing against bone with no cartilage padding between the vertebrae.

With this diagnosis came many gardening and life restrictions. There would be no more hefting 50-pound bags on my shoulders, weeding for eight hours straight, or heavy digging in the garden. Any action that involved heavier work would have to be re-learned in order to prevent further damage to my back and neck. In fact, I had to re-learn how to sit, how to stand, how to bend, and how to reach. I began a new regimen of walking one hour per day, based upon my doctor's recommendation. I did this all while living with extreme pain and worrying that my career, which is very much centered on gardening, would be over. I was devastated.

Because there is no cure for this type of osteoarthritis, most doctors work to make the victim of this condition more comfortable. As a solution for the intense pain, the doctor typically

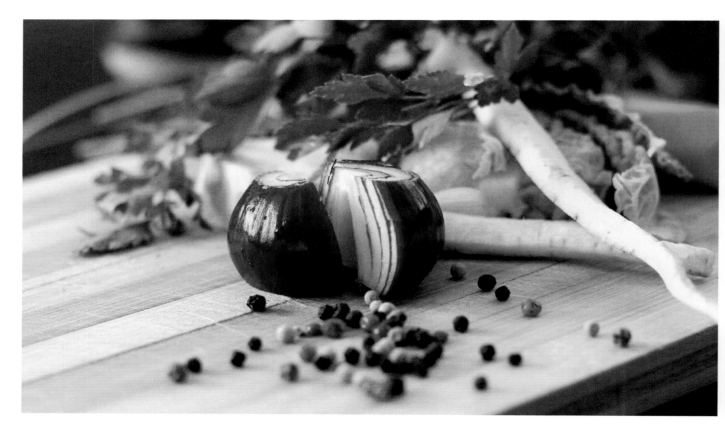

"Food is the cure," according to certified nutritionist Deepa Deshmukh, an individual who came to play a very important role in my life. Reducing inflammation in the body is possible by consuming anti-inflammatory foods such as fresh vegetables and healthy fats. Consuming a diet rich in vegetables can also help lower cholesterol and heart disease while reducing inflammation in the body.
Public Domain Pixabay.com.

suggests medicated pain therapy—drugs—combined with physical therapy. There are hundreds of types of pain medications, and many are addictive drugs that can be over-prescribed. Chief among these are opioids.

According to the National Institute on Drug Abuse, chronic pain affects more than 100 million Americans, more than one-third of the United States population. While "pain therapy" is sometimes very much needed in a patient's treatment, opioids are being over-prescribed. In the United States, the National Department of Health

and Human Services calls it "the opioid epidemic," and over $55 billion is spent annually in health and social costs related to prescription-opioid abuse. Further, $20 billion is spent in emergency departments and inpatient care for opioid poisonings. In 2014 alone, more than 240 million prescriptions were written for prescription opioids.

When considering these statistics, it became evident to me that pain medication does not cure the specific problem of chronic pain: it simply masks the symptoms. So, how could I discover a cure for my own incurable condition without using addictive medications? How could I garden, walk, and sleep more freely without pain? The answer came, at least in my mind, from an unlikely source.

FOOD AND DIET FOR WELLNESS

Chronic pain related to inflammation happens when the body elicits a localized protective response to a specific area within the body. Both doctors and physical therapists agree that in order to reduce the pain in my body, I would need to reduce the inflammation I was experiencing. Chief signs of inflammation are redness, swelling, heat, pain, and loss of joint, muscle, and organ function. Chronic inflammation can cause the following health concerns: obesity and weight gain, chronic pain, allergies, fibromyalgia, chronic bronchitis, asthma, heart disease, diabetes, arthritis, irritable bowel syndrome, peptic ulcer, certain cancers, and many more.

I met with a certified nutritionist, Deepa Deshmukh, MPH, RD, BC-ADM, CDE, who also suggested reducing inflammation as a way to reduce pain. Deepa felt that while not everyone with chronic pain has inflammation, chronic inflammation is significantly present during most chronic pain episodes. She suggested attacking the pain by reducing the inflammation with an anti-inflammatory diet, stating, "Food is the cure."

THE DIET

Before you consider a dietary change, consult with your own doctors and nutritional experts, because your personal health concerns will direct the exercise and diet routine you should adopt. I worked with Deepa to develop my dietary plan. First we built a daily nutritional food list based on

Top Eight Food Allergens

According to the United States Department of Agriculture, there are eight top food allergens that can cause allergic reactions and inflammation-related reactions. These eight foods account for about 90 percent of all food-related allergic reactions and are also base food sources from which many other ingredients for other foods are derived. Without an allergy test or a severe reaction such as anaphylaxis, it's hard to know if you are having a lesser-allergic reaction, such as inflammation, swelling, itching, sinus issues, and other complaints, to one of these items. Eliminating these potential allergens, at least on a temporary basis, and gradually reintroducing them can help reduce reactions and therefore inflammation.

- Milk
- Eggs
- Fish
- Crustacean shellfish
- Tree nuts
- Peanuts
- Wheat
- Soybeans

anti-inflammatory principles. Deepa gave me a dietary list to follow that included an increase of whole foods with an emphasis on no grains, no dairy, and no sugars.

Next, we focused on my body's reactions. Certain foods caused me pain and discomfort while other foods did not. How do we determine which food is making me react without my taking a formal allergy test? Our solution was to research the top eight food allergens as recommended by the federal government (see "Top Eight Food Allergens") and temporarily restrict these foods along with the basics—no dairy, no grain, no sugar—for 30 days. In order to remind myself to stay on the diet, I began using an online tracking

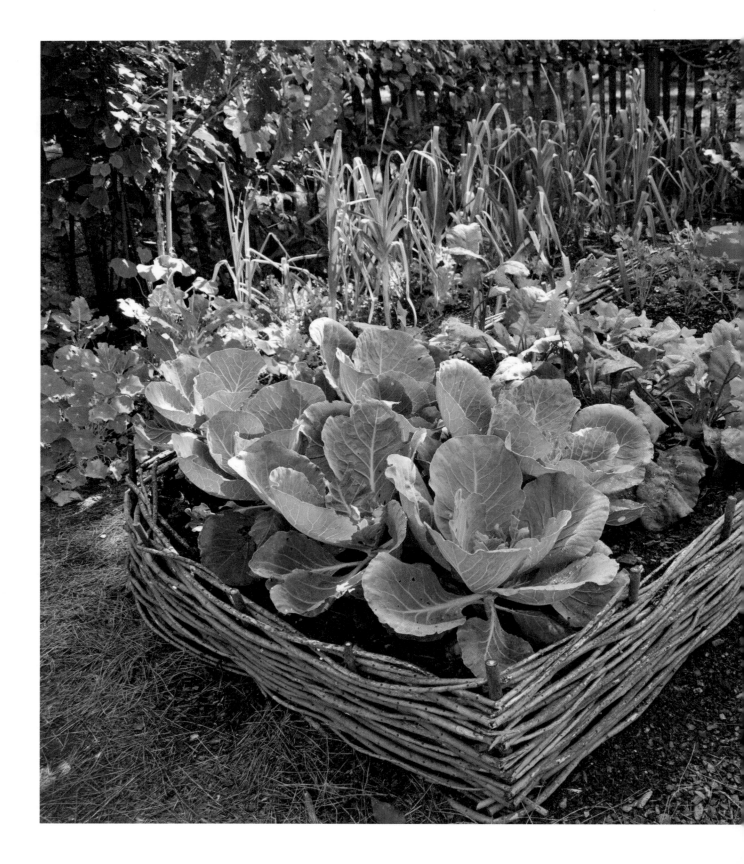

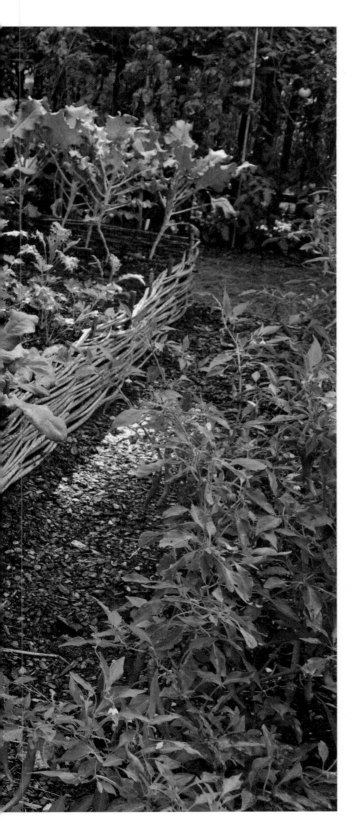

device to keep track of what I ate, sticking with Deepa's recommended daily caloric intake and strict lists. When I began the anti-inflammatory diet, I was consuming 1,200 calories per day. Deepa insisted I increase my diet by at least 300 to 400 calories per day with foods that were high in fat. She wanted me to eat more avocadoes, seeds, oils, and olives.

When I left the first office visit with Deepa, I cried. I thought I would not be able to eat anything. I thought I would be so alone. I thought I would fail. I thought the diet was ridiculous and entirely too difficult. I thought I would continue to have extreme chronic pain. And I most certainly thought that 30 days would last forever.

ANTI-INFLAMMATORY FOOD

What happened next was shocking: the diet was easier than I thought it would be. I discovered soups, meat, vegetables, herbs, and spices that were flavorful and delicious. Rather quickly, the diet began to relieve my pain without the use of additional pain medications. It also revealed how much I love vegetables. For the first time in my life, vegetables in particular began to taste great. Choosing whole vegetables and whole foods over processed foods became an easier and easier choice as time went on. With the elimination of heavy carbohydrates and sugars from my diet, all

Large quantities of vegetables and herbs can be grown in small garden spaces using raised beds or containers. Planting herbs and vegetables closely together makes it possible to supplement your diet with fresh food at a low cost even in small areas. Inexpensive growing techniques make such gardening affordable. This elevated bed cost the gardener very little and was made from branch cuttings and compost. *Photo taken at Chanticleer Garden.*

food had a different and better taste. This led to my growing more of my own herbs and vegetables and combining these fresh garden foods with the groceries I found at the supermarket.

As I continued down my anti-inflammatory journey, food became my primary thought every day. How to eat food, where to find the best food, and how to afford food captured my thoughts. Most significantly, I explored the vitamin content of the foods I was growing organically at home. (Later in this book, I explore which fruits, herbs, and vegetables have the most vitamin content so that you can better determine the nutritional value of the foods you grow.)

With my diagnosis came a lot of unsolicited advice from friends, most of it founded in myth with no scientific evidence to back up the claims. Soaking raisins in gin and consuming a dozen of them per day does nothing for arthritis swelling, yet it is a common online claim. Drinking cider vinegar is not scientifically proven to ease pain, yet it is splashed all over the internet as a solution.

Healthy fats include avocadoes, avocado oil, nuts, nut butter, hummus, seeds, olive oil, coconut, coconut oil, eggs, sunflower oil, and fatty fish. Combined with fresh vegetables and low-fat meats, healthy fats can help your body process foods, make you feel full after meals, protect you against heart disease, and help your body function properly. *Public Domain Pixabay.com.*

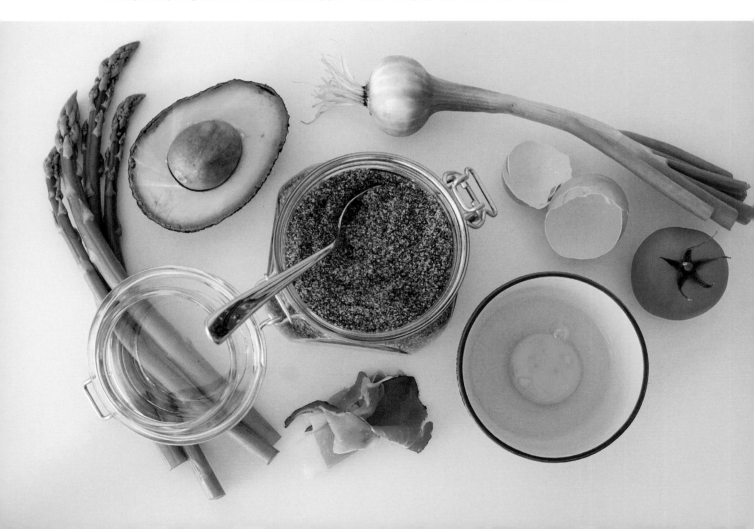

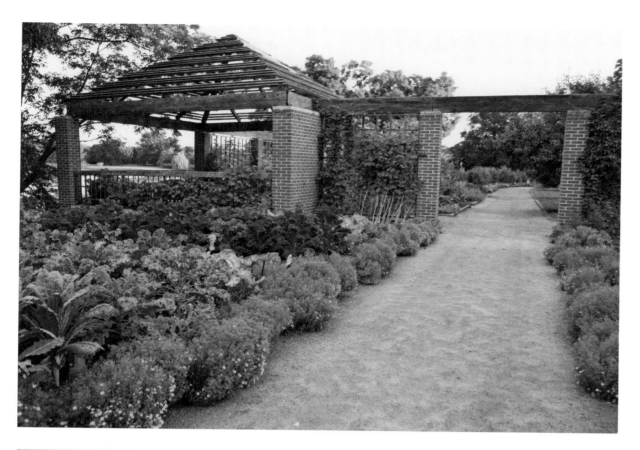

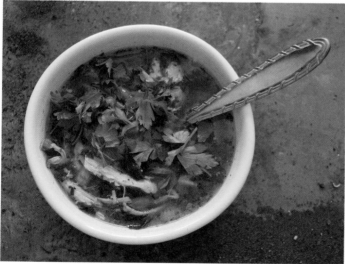

ABOVE: Landscaping with vegetables is a remarkable way to supplement a fresh food list that will contribute to an anti-inflammatory diet and contribute beauty to your gardens, walking paths, and community. Vegetables and herbs that have more color typically have more vitamin content. So, select colorful ornamental edibles for your garden for healthier harvests.

LEFT: At first I thought that a restrictive diet would make eating flavorful dishes with fresh herbs and vegetables challenging, but I soon found out that there were lots of delicious meals to be discovered that featured soups, meat, and vegetables, all seasoned with herbs and spices fresh from the garden, that were flavorful and delicious. Chicken and kale soup with parsley is extremely flavorful and one of my favorites.

WHAT IS A WELLNESS GARDEN?

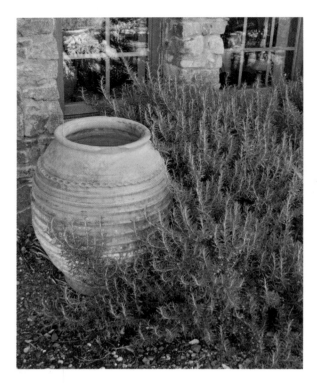

One of the true secrets to making vegetables and meats taste better is to add fresh herbs to your recipes. Grow herbs on a window sill in the winter; during the summer, incorporate them into your gardens and landscape. Your pathways will smell delicious, and you can create small garden vignettes that transform your garden into an emotionally therapeutic place that will help restore your health.

Coffee is supposed to be patently bad for arthritis, but according to studies, coffee or tea is fine. It's more likely that the flavorings, dairy, and sugar you put in the coffee are causing an issue.

Chief among these false stories is that Solanaceae vegetables from the nightshade family trigger arthritis swelling and pain. There is absolutely no formal scientific testing to corroborate this myth, yet unsubstantiated claims run rampant across the internet. In my own personal experience, I have noticed that tomatoes, peppers, tomatillo, goji berries, eggplant, and yams—all from the Solanaceae family—do not trigger my osteoarthritis pain. White potatoes, however, make me feel bloated and achy. Potatoes are a starchy carbohydrate food that is high on the glycemic index. Scientific studies have shown that a lower carbohydrate, higher fat diet decreases levels of saturated fat, lowers blood sugar, and most importantly keeps inflammation down.

The Importance of the Glycemic Index (GI)

The glycemic index (GI) is a numeric value assigned to individual foods based on how the food causes blood glucose level increases within the human body. There is significant variability in studies on specific GI results, but in general, conclusions say that certain foods are higher and other foods are lower on the GI. Higher GI foods increase our blood sugar and speed of digestion. You can make a conscious decision to consume a lower GI and carbohydrate diet in which slower, steadier digestion aids your body by reducing inflammation and leaves you less hungry between meals.

By and large, carbohydrates are good for your body, providing the energy you need for bodily processes. They help our gut bacteria digest food. But some carbohydrates have a higher GI score. According to the Harvard Medical School Health Publication, higher glycemic index diets may stimulate inflammation because they cause higher and more rapid increases in blood glucose levels. In a Brazilian university study at the Instituto Federal de Educação, it was shown that a low glycemic index diet also reduced body fat and attenuated inflammatory and metabolic responses in patients with Type 2 diabetes. Similarly, studies on obese adults who consumed a lower GI diet showed those people experienced a significant decrease in cardiac-related inflammation. Patients who were able to reduce inflammation were often able to help reduce their chronic pain.

With this information in hand, I worked to develop a lower carbohydrate food list that might have consistently lower GI scores that I could grow in my garden. I began growing my own lower carbohydrate foods and considering my reactions to them. My lowest pain levels and bloating reactions came from low-carbohydrate, high-vitamin vegetables such as swiss chard, bok choy, spinach, and arugula.

REINTRODUCING FOOD

Once I dedicated myself to the diet for 30 days, I fell into a habit of eating that helped me realize that the plan was more than an anti-inflammatory diet: it was also the start of a healthier permanent lifestyle. Deepa held my hand every step of the way and encouraged me to continue my daily walking and gardening, along with the diet. Once I had surpassed the 30-day mark, I began gradually reintroducing certain foods to expand my options.

Reintroducing foods after a 30-day period of clean eating enabled me to find which foods clearly caused a reaction such as pain, sinusitis, asthma, bloating, diarrhea, gas, constipation, heartburn, or swelling. When reintroducing foods, it is important to introduce only one new food about once per week and only consume a small amount of that food. Gauge your body's reaction. I discovered that even within the same family of foods, some caused

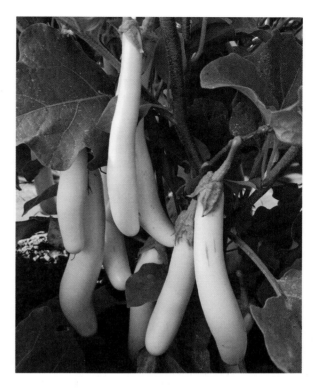

Solanaceae vegetables from the nightshade family have not been scientifically proven to trigger arthritis pain. These plants include tomatoes, peppers, tomatillo, goji berries, eggplant, potatoes, and yams. Plants like this Japanese white eggplant ('Gretel', which was an All-American Selections winner in 2016) are only a call for worry if you are specifically allergic or sensitive to members of the nightshade family. Cautious sampling or blood testing with a doctor's supervision can determine if you should eliminate specific vegetables due to allergy.

strong reactions and others produced lesser or no reactions. For example, I cannot eat lobster, yet I can eat scallops. I cannot eat peanuts, yet I can eat almonds. I cannot have most dairy, yet I can have a dairy-based oil called ghee. I can eat almost every vegetable, herb, and spice. I discovered these things by trying one new food per week and working closely with my nutritionist.

GROW AND EXERCISE FOR WELLNESS

Of course, growing and eating fresh vegetables are part of a wellness lifestyle. But a physical connection to the garden—regularly touching plants and soil, simply enjoying the beauty of the garden—also plays an important role. Since the Middle Ages, medicinal and aesthetically beautiful gardens have been grown to provide that restorative experience to gardeners and visitors alike.

Consider this: modern science has shown that simply touching soil can provide a mood boost. *Mycobacterium vaccae*, a particular bacterium strain found in soil, has been shown in the Bristol University study ("Identification of an Immune-Responsive Mesolimbocortical Serotonergic System: Potential Role in Regulation of Emotional Behavior," by Christopher Lowry et al., published online on March 28, 2007, in *Neuroscience*) to trigger the release of serotonin in people who experience direct contact with soil. This connection decreases stress anxiety and elevates mood. While the mood-elevating effect can last beyond the initial exposure, according to further studies at Sage Colleges, one must be regularly reconnected with soil to retain the effect, which can last up to three weeks after exposure.

Gardening also decreases cortisol, a stress response hormone, according to a study done by Agnes Vandenberg of the Wageningen University and Research Center in The Netherlands. Therapeutic gardening began catching on for people who suffer depression and post-traumatic stress disorder because being in a garden has the unique ability to improve a person's feelings about him- or herself and the world. Seeing yourself in a better light builds confidence and helps with emotionally unstable situations. This, in turn, can help a person feel less depressed and have less anxiety.

This has been very true on my own property—gardening has changed my attitude. I find myself feeling upbeat and positive when I spend more time tending plants. Exposure to the garden on a regular basis has become a part of my osteoarthritis physical therapy. I have learned that there is no need to overstrain yourself in the garden: with a little planning, you can use the proper tools and elevate beds so you can sit or stand while gardening. There is evidence that gardening can help you in other

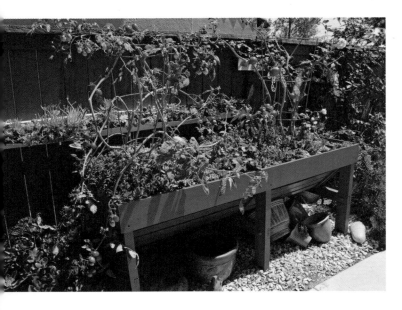

In San Diego, California, I met up with Laura Eubanks at her home garden. Tucked along a fence in a small side yard is this charming elevated bed that contained a mix of succulents and vegetables. Most vegetables are surprisingly low in carbohydrates and also have lower glycemic index scores. So, tuck them in with your traditional plantings as Laura has done.

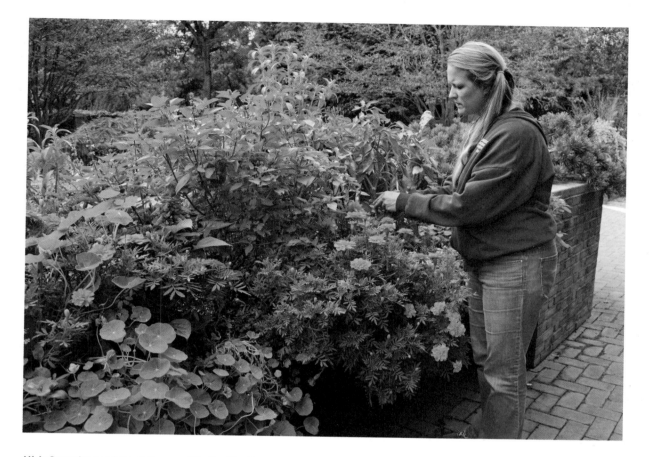

Alicia Green is one of the designers of the Buehler Enabling Garden at the Chicago Botanic Garden. Her design goal has been to elevate beds in order to create a more comfortable gardening space for people who suffer with chronic pain and other conditions that prevent them from gardening on the ground. These elevated beds are great for growing flowers, vegetables, and vines.

therapeutic ways beyond emotional boosts and moderate exercise.

For example, in a 2011 study published in the *New England Journal of Medicine*, children were less likely to develop asthma if they grew up on a traditional farm where they spent time gardening and regularly playing in the dirt. These types of studies and experiences lead theorists to redefine horticultural therapy. Originally, it was thought that gardening was particularly therapeutic

because of the physical exercise involved. With the latest research on healing landscapes and horticultural therapy, it is clear that planting an organic vegetable garden (whether it be in ground, in elevated beds, or in container gardens) and then nurturing and harvesting it, you are also harvesting better mental health simply by putting your hands in the garden soil regularly.

Clearly, growing is important, but having that regular exposure to nature and the outside world

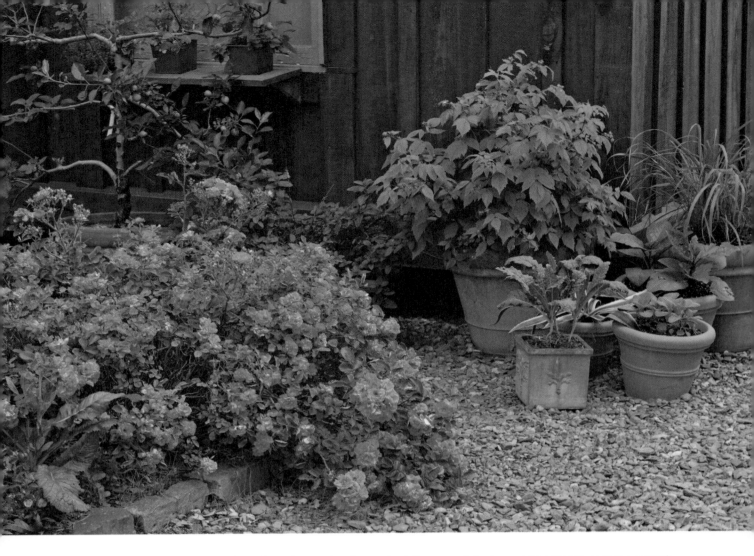

Using elevated beds, living walls, and container gardens to grow food, flowers, and plants can make a big difference in a person's well-being. Touching soil and nurturing living things has been scientifically proven to improve mood and help one's wellness outlook. This little garden niche was discovered behind a garden shed on P. Allen Smith's Moss Mountain Farm in Arkansas.

is critical and could be significantly influential on your mental state. Walking in the woods where you can see trees or along the beach where you can see the ocean and native grasses have been proven to have a positive effect on your brain. Researchers discovered, in a groundbreaking study done by the University of Illinois Landscape and Human Health Laboratory, that children living in the inner city have a greater risk of academic underachievement, juvenile delinquency, teenage pregnancy, and many other issues when deprived of contact with nature.

The study went on to reveal that, on average, the greener the view is from a girl's home, the better she can concentrate. Better concentration means she is better at inhibiting impulses and the more able she is to delay gratification. This means that exposure to nature is more likely to generate a self-disciplined mindset, which is an important personal trait in a stressful world. If a girl has strong self-discipline, she is more likely to do well in school and in life, while avoiding unhealthy or risky behaviors.

The same team from the University of Illinois conducted an additional study on aggression. This study discovered that contact with vegetation reduces mental fatigue. The research was done in a setting and population with comparatively high rates of aggression: inner-city urban public housing residents. This research shows that after studying 145 adult women, "Levels of aggression and violence were significantly lower among individuals who had some nearby nature outside their apartments than among their counterparts who lived in barren conditions." In other words, simply having a minimal view of a tree from an apartment window helped reduce aggression.

Everyone can be more emotionally healthy with regular exposure to nature. Gardening, walking,

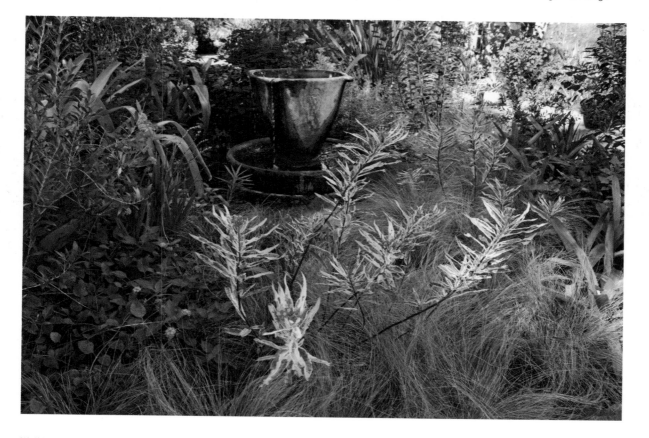

Walking in gardens such as this Teacup Garden at Chanticleer near Philadelphia can be truly inspirational. Each plant has been placed to reveal an artistic view. Artistry in the garden is an important part of the horticultural experience, as it immerses the human spirit and inspires the gardener to grow more than vegetables and herbs. Growing a better self is a part of the wellness garden lifestyle.

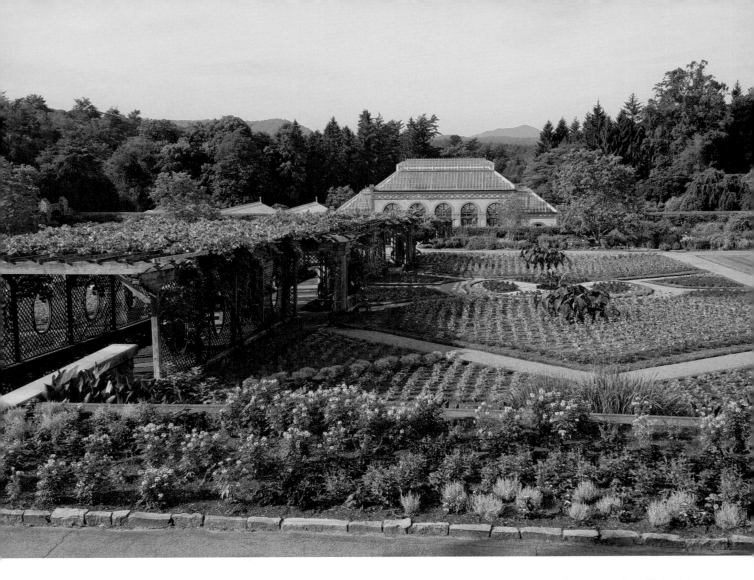

Whether you live in an urban area or in the country, it is possible to jump into nature to garden and experience nature by visiting parks and gardens. In a lovely valley in the rolling mountains of Asheville, North Carolina, you can find Biltmore Estate's amazing property, which is filled with gardens and natural areas. Biltmore's Walled Garden is a delight: it merges landscape design, perennial plantings, and walking paths beneath the glass and brick architecture of the Biltmore Conservatory. This urban garden is a lovely place to connect with the natural world and a health-minded garden.

and being active while outdoors with a specific goal of increasing your physical movement can also improve your health. No matter your physical level of mobility, being outdoors and in contact with gardens and nature helps you.

LIVING THE WELLNESS LIFESTYLE EVERY DAY

There is an old expression that taking the first step toward a goal is always the most difficult. I have been inspired by actor Will Smith's

24

The Results

On any day that I am able, I step out into nature and I garden. Every day I am able, I walk. Every day, I try to eat freshly grown vegetables and good foods. Every day is a journey toward wellness. Throughout this lifestyle change and journey, I have noticed changes in myself. And now, finally, the effects have become clear, and they are positively amazing.

- Within four days of beginning the diet, my pain reduced significantly—by approximately 40 percent in my estimation.
- Within four weeks, my blood pressure went down 40 points and I went off blood-pressure medicines.
- Within eight weeks, most of my menopause symptoms went away.
- By 12 weeks, I noticed the pain I still had was down more than half what it was when I was diagnosed.
- Within 18 weeks, I went off all extended prescription medications for my asthma.

- My mood improved significantly, and I stopped suffering winter-induced seasonal affective disorder.
- After 12 months, I averaged a largely significant reduction in pain—by approximately 80 percent in my estimation
- Allergy and asthma symptoms were greatly reduced.
- While the diet—particularly eating garden fresh vegetables—is very important to inflammation reduction, it has been equally important to stay active and move my body daily. All this is the wellness lifestyle—gardening, walking, diet, and food.

belief that there is power in speaking things into existence. When you say something into being, your subconscious allows you to make it achievable because you motivate yourself to confidence. As Will Smith said, "The first step is you have to say that you can."

Chronic pain ruled my life, but I took control of my body and lifestyle in order to reduce pain and consistently feel better in every aspect of my life. If you feel your wellness plan is not where it should be, only you can take the first step to change it. Do you have inflammation or pain like I have, or do you want to make a step toward wellness? It can be as easy as making that first appointment with your doctor and nutritionist. They are your guides toward better health. Get second opinions, read books, and

learn what the best fit is for you and your family from a diet and exercise perspective. Change your lifestyle for a healthier outlook.

No matter how small or large your growing area is, you can garden. Whether you have no pain or health problems or suffer from extreme pain and in need of a doctor's supervision, you can improve your lifestyle. Each chapter of this book gives tips and ideas for you to learn how to make your garden a healing place—both from a nutritional and food-growing perspective and also from a relaxing and therapeutic perspective.

By committing yourself to wellness and to live more mindfully, you make a choice every single day on how you want to live, eat, move, and travel your life path.

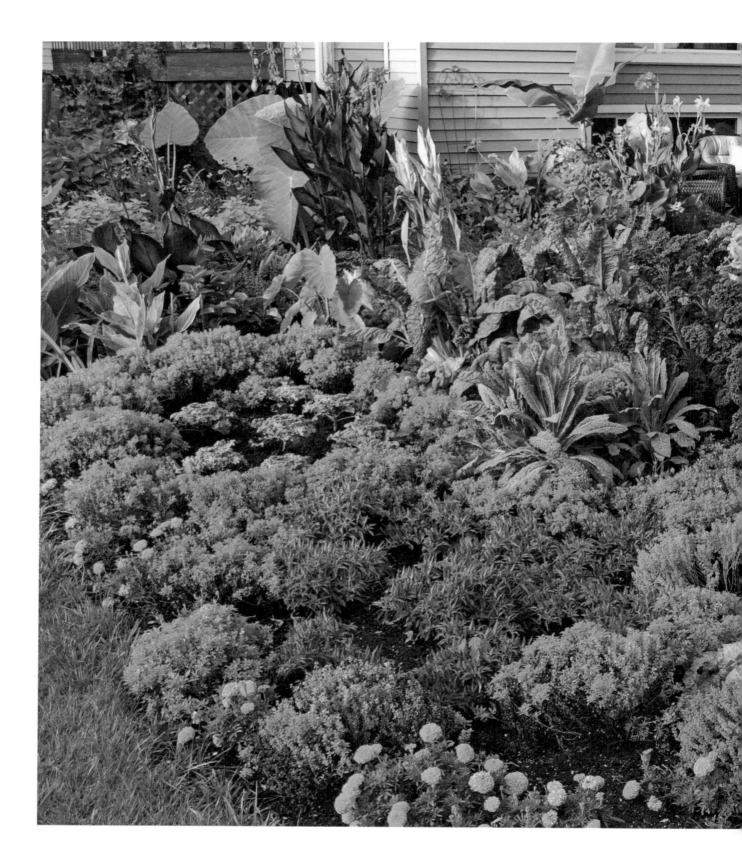

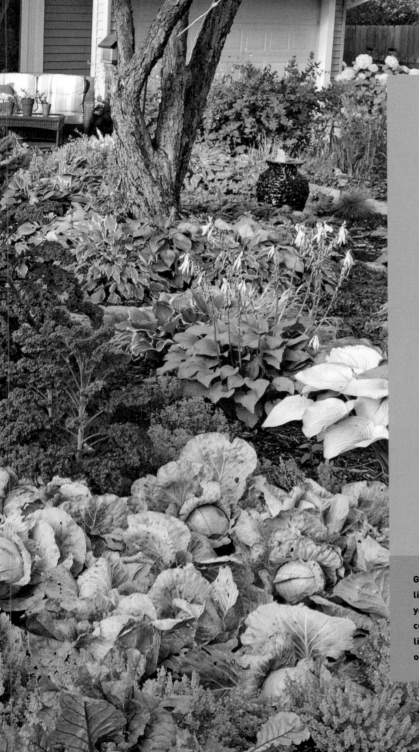

PART I

GROWING THE WELLNESS DIET & LIFESTYLE

Growing a whole-food diet garden for your wellness lifestyle can fit into whatever your space allows. Whether you have an urban balcony, suburban front lawn, or country farm, gardening can make a difference in your life and the lives of your neighbors. Here is my front-lawn ornamental edible vegetable garden.

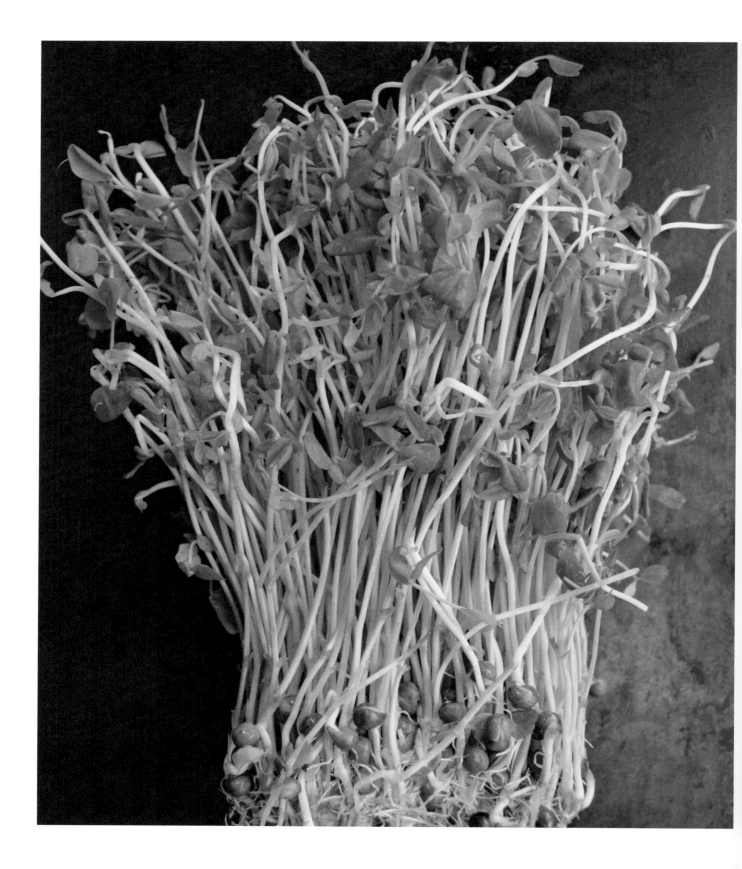

1

GROWING THE WELLNESS DIET

FIND WHOLE FOODS

ONCE I DISCOVERED that restricting sugary carbohydrates and dairy foods could stimulate my taste for vegetables and herbs, I began an all-out effort to learn how to find the fresh whole foods that gave the taste and nutrient explosion I was wanted at every meal. According to the book *Food as Medicine Everyday*, "The standard American diet . . . is highly processed and nutrient-poor." Indeed, the typical shopping market is full of processed foods. Whole food, on the other hand, has been refined as little as possible and has very few additives and artificial substances. Foods that are "whole" usually have more fiber, have less of the bad fats and processed cane sugar, and often come in their original fruit or vegetable form.

Finding foods that contain fewer chemicals is simple: when you are able to choose, always go for the most natural choice. For example, a whole apple is less processed, has more fiber, and is fresher than a jar of applesauce to which high fructose corn syrup and other chemicals have been added. In your quest to find foods that are

OPPOSITE: Living pea tendrils and microgreens possess an exceptionally high number of nutrients per calorie and are an excellent whole food choice. Pea tendrils sometimes come with leaves attached, while at other times they will be more sprout-like. Chop pea tendrils and leaves, then use them on salads and in stir frying as a vegetable similar to spinach. It has a slightly sweet taste with a nutty undertone.

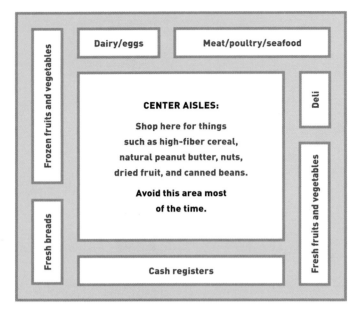

LEFT: "Shop the outside aisles of the grocery store," recommends the Massachusetts Health and Human Services organization. In this chart you can see that the whole food items such as fresh and frozen whole fruits and vegetables, eggs, meat, seafood, and poultry are typically located on the perimeter aisles of a grocery store. Some healthy whole foods such as nuts, nut butter, dried fruit, and canned or dried beans can be found in the center aisles (along with processed foods that might not be as healthful). Shop carefully and with an eye to health.

OPPOSITE: Gardening in the ground is the most basic form of gardening. All you need is good soil, regular water, and a bit of sunshine to create abundant herbs, vegetables, and flowers. Here is a lovely view of a cold-weather crop ripening in very late summer before the cool weather sets in at the Chicago Botanic Garden. *Photo taken at Chicago Botanic Garden.*

healthy, try to consume foods that are raw, fresh, and in their original form. Fresh garlic in bulb form is a whole food. Canned minced garlic is not a whole food as it could contain garlic, water, citric acid, and sodium benzoate or another artificial ingredient. Choose whole and fresh over processed for a healthier diet.

Generally speaking, whole foods are more likely to be found around the perimeter of a supermarket. When walking the center aisles of a supermarket you will find mostly packaged goods. Many of these packaged foods contain excessive amounts of chemical additives, refined sugars, and food colorings. They are usually over-processed. An anti-inflammatory diet starts with whole foods, not heavily processed foods.

During the winter months in some states, cold weather limits gardening. So, you need to be aware of where in your local store you can find healthier whole foods when you can't grow them yourself.

FIND FIBER

Fiber is the part of plants that we do not digest, but it still benefits us as it moves through our digestive systems helping to remove carcinogens, lower cholesterol levels, control blood sugar levels, prevent cancer, and essentially keep our systems moving in a healthy way. Most people perceive fiber as being "whole grains," which can be an important part of a whole foods diet. However, if your nutritionist or doctor has recommended an anti-inflammatory elimination diet with no bread or grain, where do you get your fiber?

According to the Mayo Clinic Nutrition and Healthy Eating resource, the best fiber choices are fruits, vegetables, beans, peas, legumes, nuts, and seeds as well as whole-grain products. The Mayo Clinic suggests women have 21 to 25 grams of fiber a day and men should aim for 30 to 38 grams a day. In a study done by the US Department of Agriculture, the average daily fiber intake of an American

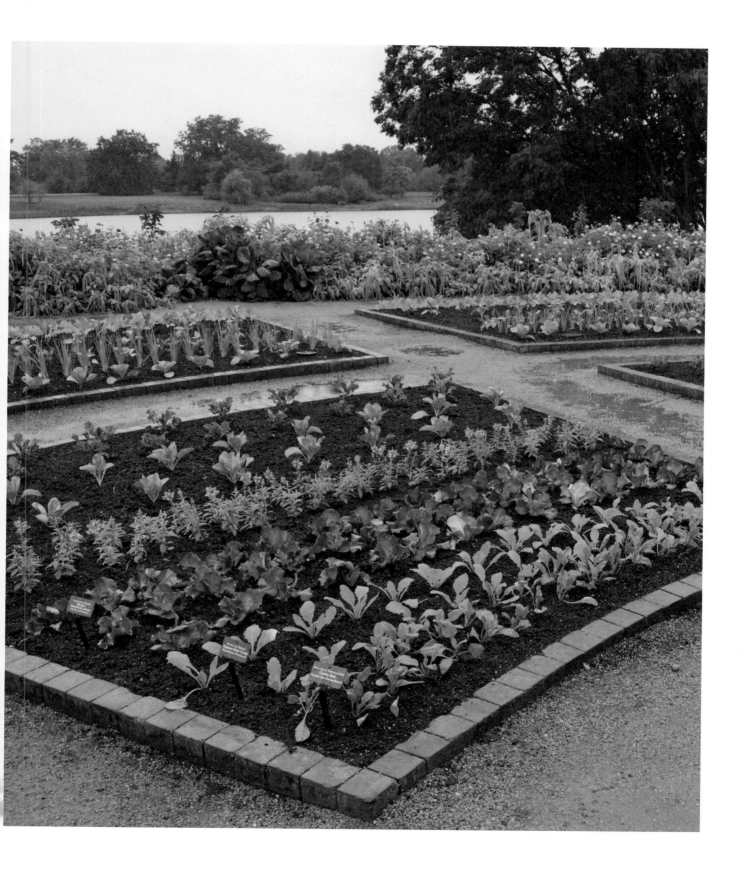

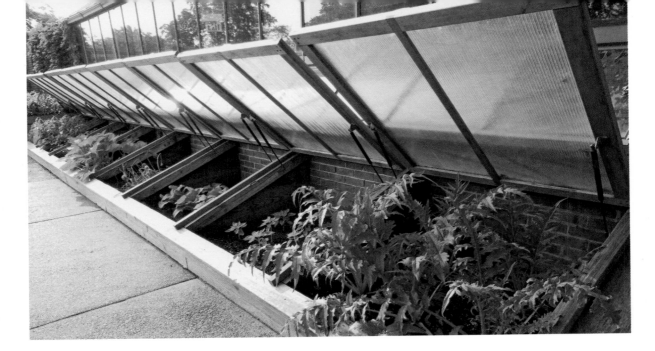

Cold frames, such as these at the Chicago Botanic Garden, can help extend the growing season for your garden for year-round herb- and vegetable-growing convenience. Typically, a cold frame has four sides and a removable glass or plastic lid that allows light to come in and keep plants warm and alive without artificial heat or electricity in colder climes. *Photo taken at Chicago Botanic Garden.*

was approximately 16 grams per day, which is significantly lower than the recommended minimum. Finding a way to increase your fiber can decrease your risk of disease.

Fruits, vegetables, and beans are great sources of fiber and are considered excellent choices for an anti-inflammatory diet. Increasing your fiber intake by growing and consuming high-fiber foods can make you feel better. One cup of strawberries, blackberries, and raspberries have about 8 grams of dietary fiber and are remarkably easy to grow. An avocado has between 10 and 13 grams of fiber. Many lentils and beans have over 10 grams of fiber. Generally speaking, whole raw fruits and vegetables are some of the easiest ways to add fiber to your diet, and you can get them right outside your door if you grow a garden.

Planning a garden to include fruits, herbs, and vegetables rich in high fiber and color is a great way to provide a balanced diet, but also to reduce spending. Growing your own whole food year round can supplement visits to the grocery with fresher and healthier choices.

TRY FALL AND WINTER GARDENING

Part of your plan to find and incorporate more whole foods in your diet might be deciding how you will grow herbs and vegetables through the late fall and winter. If you live in a warmer gardening zone, it is possible to harvest a large range of fresh vegetables all year long. Should you live in the colder north, you might find it more difficult to grow once it frosts regularly or when you have 6 to 12 inches of snow on the ground.

Cold-Hardy Vegetable List

Below are two vegetable lists that feature herbs and vegetables that can grow during colder seasons as recommended by cold season garden expert Niki Jabbour from SavvyGardening.com.

These are vegetables that can be grown and harvested through winter in USDA garden zone 4 and higher if protected from frost and heavy snow with covers.

Plant will typically last through early winter, with a harvest date no later than the end of December.

- Arugula
- Beets
- Bok choy*
- Broccoli*
- Brussels sprouts
- Cabbage*
- Carrots
- Collard greens
- Jerusalem artichokes
- Kale
- Kohlrabi*
- Leeks
- Mustard greens
- Parsnips
- Radishes
- Rapini*
- Rutabaga
- Spinach
- Swiss chard
- Turnips

Food Crops that Overwinter

These vegetables can generally overwinter without protection and provide a very early spring crop in USDA garden zones 4 and higher.

- Carrots
- Chives
- Garlic
- Kale
- Leeks
- Onions
- Oregano
- Parsnips
- Sage
- Thyme

However, there are creative solutions. Niki Jabbour, author of the book *The Year-Round Vegetable Gardener*, has inspired me to expand the growing season through winter for the crops that appreciate colder temperatures. While it can be challenging to grow vegetables through northern winters, it is not impossible, and it will certainly contribute to a healthier diet. Niki's techniques and ideas for winter growing include using cold frames and covered hoop tunnels as protective shelters from the snow.

Good planning is important for fall or winter growing. Build a special cover for your cold-weather vegetable crop before the cold sets in. During heavy snows, it is necessary to tighten up hoop tunnel covers to prevent the plastic covers or frost cloths from touching and crushing the plants. Cold frames are also a fantastic place to acclimate seedlings grown indoors in the spring.

GROW "FAST FOOD"

Many of the colorful leafy vegetables that are high in fiber and nutrition are very easy to grow and also grow surprisingly fast. This enables you to produce lots of food quickly. Leafy greens, living pea tendrils, microgreens and shoots, spinach, and radishes are outstanding food choices to grow in a small space. This makes them smart choices for urban balcony or patio growing as they can be grown closely together in tight spaces such as living walls, container gardens, small elevated beds, or even on a sunny windowsill.

Choosing to plant fast-growing vegetables means that you can harvest the vegetables sooner and that, in turn, enables you to replant vegetables for a second, third, or fourth crop throughout the season. You can have a constant source of fresh food by planting these fast-growing crops in alternating weeks: plant every two weeks

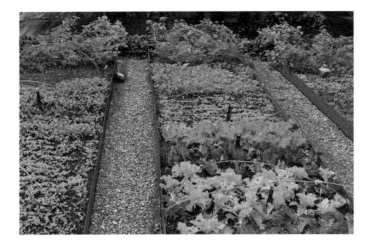

Fast-growing microgreens and leafy vegetables such as these found at Chef Rick Bayless's home are easy to grow from seed. Cover the vegetables with netting to prevent pests from bothering the plantings. Pick the vegetables as needed to use in salads, toppings, garnishes, and lettuce wraps.

throughout the spring and summer, and you'll always have fresh food at your fingertips.

Microgreens are particularly important whole foods. In a recent study done by the US Department of Agriculture, researchers discovered that microgreens have highly concentrated

Vegetables that Grow Quickly

Fast-growing vegetables such as the ones listed below produce quick results; you could harvest in 30 days or less.

- Arugula
- Beet greens
- Chard
- Green onions
- Kale
- Lettuces
- Microgreens
- Mustard greens
- Radish
- Spinach
- Sprouts
- Sunflower shoots
- Tatsoi
- Turnip greens

phytonutrient-per-calorie values. Phytonutrients are found in fruits and vegetables. They are different from vitamins in that they are not essential for keeping a human being alive, yet studies show they may be important in preventing disease and keeping your body functioning healthily. Some phytonutrient-filled microgreens can be grown in less than two weeks, which definitely makes them fast garden-to-table food. Many microgreens have increased levels of color and flavor, so they taste as good as they look.

BUY AND GROW LOCAL

Most people do not grow *all* the food they need for their family. Depending on the size of your household, you might only have a small area in which to grow, certainly not enough space to grow food year-round to supply all your food requirements. In this case, planning an organic food garden as a supplement makes sense. For example, growing foods that are too expensive in the market can be grown for less money at home. If you cannot find certain fresh vegetables you would like in the organic section of your grocer or local farm market, you can provide them yourself.

Fruits and vegetables we find in the grocery stores are often grown and sold specifically for their shelf life. Many varieties of apples are stored between 6 to 12 months before they are sold on the market. Carrots are harvested, processed, and then sold up to 9 months later. Tomatoes, peppers, and many other vegetables are harvested while still green in order to ripen on the shelves. Transportation of fruits and vegetables can last five days between locations. This type of harvesting, transportation, and storage can degrade the vitamin content of the fruits, herbs, and vegetables we consume. If fruits and vegetables are handled gently and stored at a higher humidity with refrigeration, there is a stronger likelihood that more nutrients are maintained. As a consumer we should be asking the question, "Precisely when was this fruit or vegetable harvested?" This will help us determine how nutritionally sound our food might be.

When you shop at community supported agriculture co-ops (CSAs), fruit stands, farmers markets, and even at your grocery produce department, search for the "grown local" signs and ask questions about how long ago your food was harvested. It tells a story about the health of your produce.

But the very best guarantee of freshness is to grow your own organic herbs, fruits, and vegetables and pick that produce at the height of ripeness. Then you know you are capturing the highest nutritional value, heightened color, and better flavor.

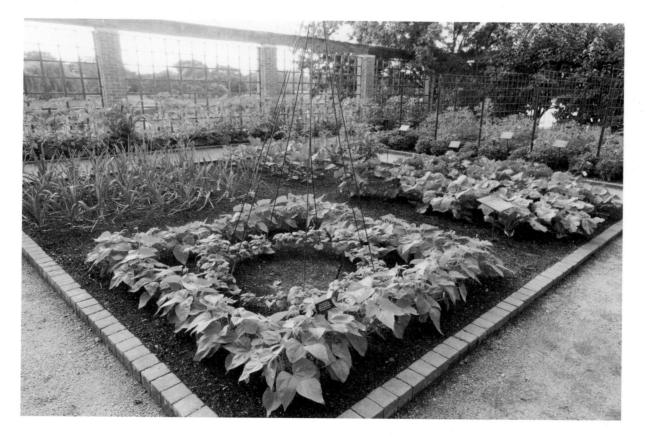

Beans are high in fiber and nutritional value, so they make a wonderful choice to grow in an organic whole foods garden. In the spring, build a pea tower for the pea plants to climb and surround the tower with bean plants. These plants are growing in close quarters, but are easily harvested throughout the season due to the tower's support. *Photo taken at Chicago Botanic Garden.*

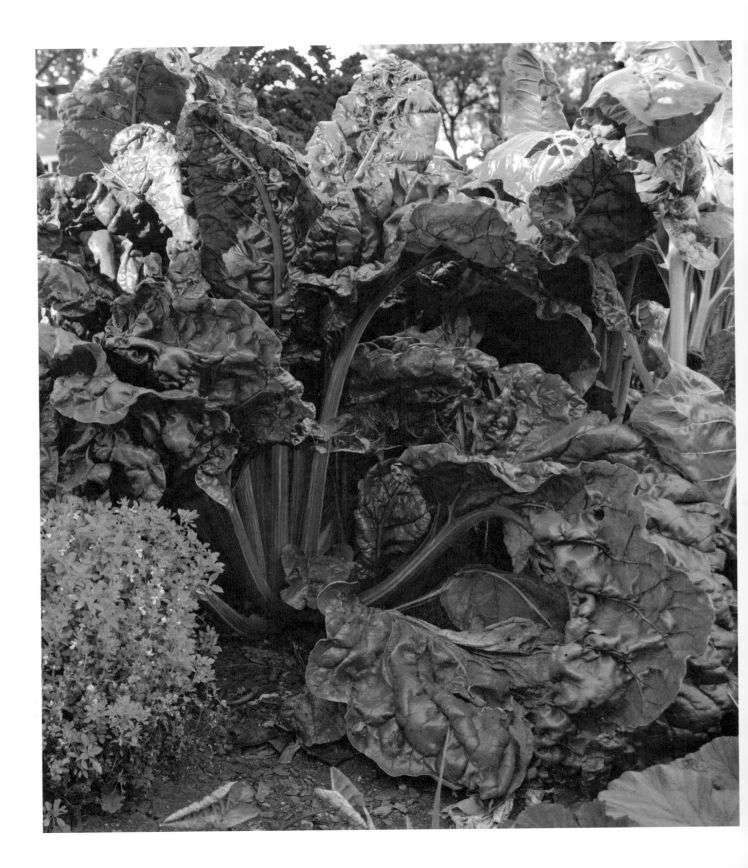

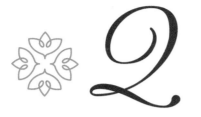

ORGANIC GARDENING BASICS FOR IN-GROUND GARDENS

WHAT IS IT that makes some people appear to have an amazing green thumb, sprouting plants wherever they plant them, while others seem to lack that skill? It is not magic. Mostly it is the understanding that a plant consistently needs three basic things to grow well: **quality soil, water, and sunlight.**

Each variety of plant has its own unique soil, water, and sunlight requirements. Some plants like shade, while other plants prefer sun. Some plants love drier soil, while other plants love wet feet. Understanding the basic requirements of each plant by reading the seed packages and plant tags can help you have more success with your plants.

OPPOSITE: Perennial, annual, herb, and vegetable plants can grow to large sizes when given the proper soil conditions with adequate water and sunlight. Swiss chard, in particular, has beautiful color and lots of nutrients, making it a great whole food choice for a healthier diet.

BUILD BETTER SOIL

Good organic soil is the secret to success: it is the most significant ingredient in the garden. If your plant has strong roots, then it will be able to survive through harsh conditions such as drought and disease. Healthy soil equals stronger roots. To better understand your soil, it is important to test its content. Soil tests can discover poisons in the soil, or simply indicate pH and fertility components. Order test kits online, purchase them at a local

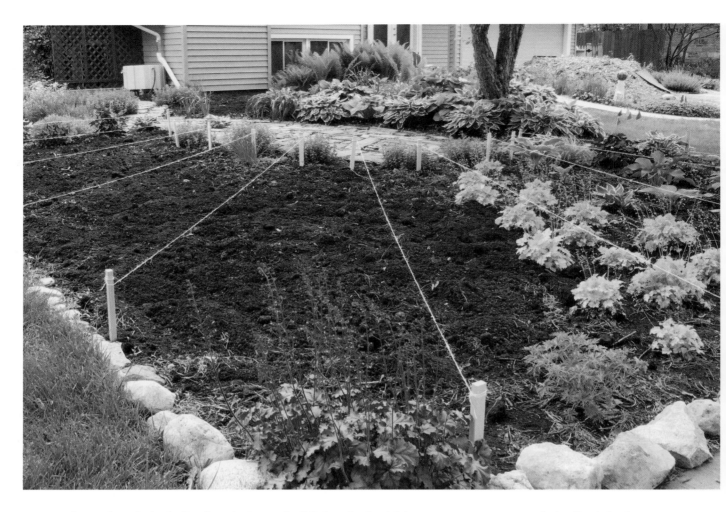

Success in gardening is often dependent on good soil. Before planting, it is important to prepare your garden's soil and plan the garden layout. Using stakes and string can help you lay out a garden configuration. Once the garden is planted, consider mulching the beds to help hold moisture in the soil where it can benefit your plant roots.

garden center, or contact your local university extension office for testing through their facilities.

If you purchase a kit, its instructions will likely direct you to send soil in to a laboratory for testing. To gather a section, simply dig a core sample out from about 12 inches beneath the soil. Do this in several locations around your garden. When you get the results, you will be able to determine what soil amendments (if any) are needed in specific area for the specific plants you are growing.

While your soil test will help you determine what type of soil amendment you need, whether you have sandy, clay, loam, or silt, adding organic matter is almost always the best way to help expand and recover your soil's microbial growth. Your soil is alive with millions of microbes that promote strong root systems. Improving the soil annually with organic matter such as compost, leaf mold, rotted manure, dried grass clippings, and chopped leaves can help build that strong system.

After you have amended your soil with organic matter, you might also consider fertilizing your plants. Adding organic matter to your soil encourages less use of other fertilizers, which is much better for the environment. But if you do feel the need to fertilize, and soil tests indicate fertilizer is needed, try to use organic fertilizers. Organic fertilizers are most likely to come from minerals, plants, or animals and have varying N-P-K (nitrogen, phosphorus, potassium) values. Note: Too much fertilizer is worse than no fertilizer at all, so research carefully before adding.

MAKE YOUR OWN COMPOST

Adding compost to your soil is a wonderful natural amendment because it helps build a more complicated microbial structure in the soil. Food scraps, yard clippings, and shredded newspaper can be transformed into rich fodder that will help you grow your whole food diet. Even better, composting is very easy, and making your own soil amendments saves you money.

To make compost, simply alternate even layers of "greens" and "browns." Greens are nitrogen-rich materials; browns are carbon-rich materials. (Examples of browns and greens are listed on page 42.) You can build simple compost piles directly on the ground or purchase bins or a turning composter. Never include meat, fats, dairy, or any animal product in your pile or it will begin to smell and attract

Continued on page 42

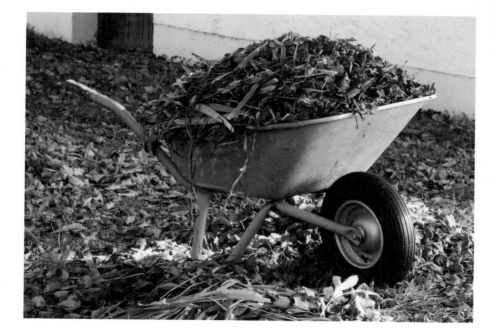

Leaves and yard waste can make excellent compost. Do not use leaves from diseased plants to make your compost, or the condition will persist in your soil and plants.

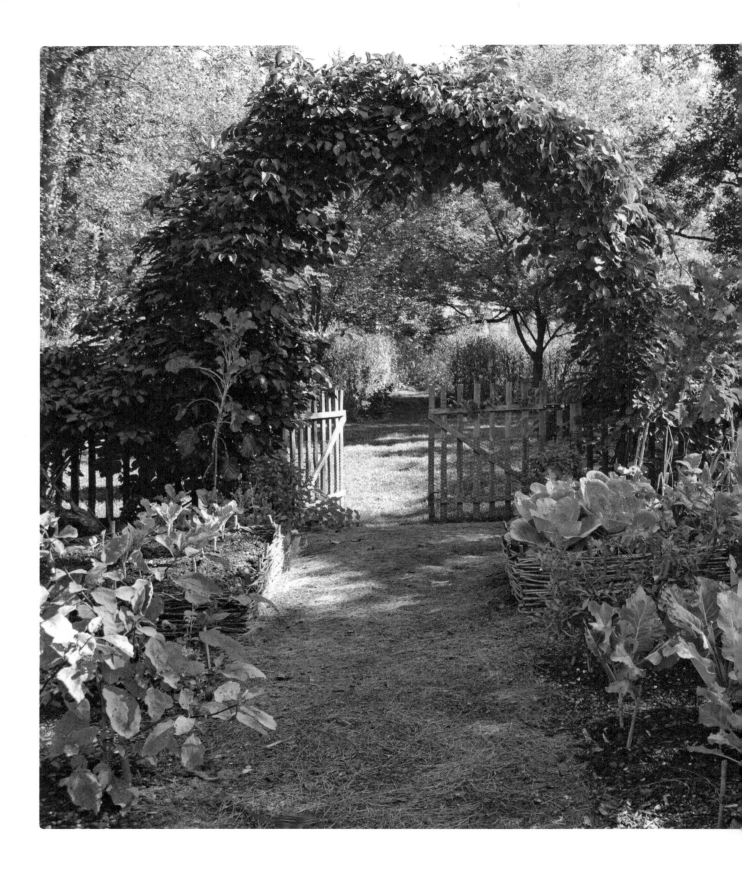

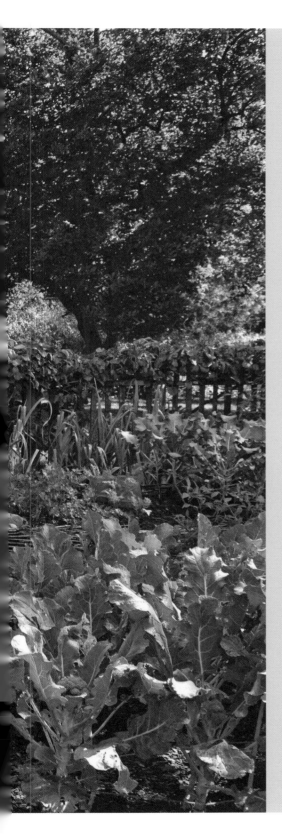

WHAT IS THE DIFFERENCE BETWEEN ORGANIC, HEIRLOOM, HYBRID, AND GMO?

What is organic? Organic foods and plants are produced using organic farming methods that do not have modern synthetic inputs like artificial pesticides and chemical fertilizers. Organic foods are not processed using industrial solvents, irradiation, or chemical food additives and do not contain genetically modified organisms (more on GMOs below). Organic foods are labeled "organic" at the grocery store and on seed packets. In other words, they are free of artificial chemical additives in any process from seed to table and are labeled as such.

What is an heirloom plant? An heirloom plant is a variety that was grown by previous generations of gardeners but is not used in today's large-scale modern agriculture. Most specifically, the plants must keep their traits uniformly through open pollination. There are varying opinions, but some say heirlooms are more than 100 years old, while others say 50 years old. Most use World War II as a dateline, saying that plant varieties developed before World War II with non-hybridization techniques are considered heirlooms. Some heirloom seed varieties are labeled "heirloom" and some are not; it's up to you to research and know the varieties in the market.

What is a hybrid plant? Hybrid plants are produced by plant breeders who engineer new varieties of plants deliberately by combining preferred or desirable characteristics of the parent plants. Hybridizing is a labor-intensive process that can be done in the field or in a laboratory and involves selecting specific plants, then removing the pollen-bearing anthers of the female plants so that only pollen from the selected male plants can be pollinated. Pollen is then manually transferred to the female plant. New plants must be cross-pollinated one generation at a time. These plants grow to full size, then develop seeds. Those seeds will not necessarily produce plants that look or produce flowers, leaves, or food like the hybrid parents, but instead, might grow a unique plant.

What is GMO? GMO is an abbreviation for "genetically modified organisms." GMOs are plants created through the gene splicing techniques of genetic engineering or biotechnology. This is an experimental technology that merges DNA from different species, creating combinations of plant, animal, bacterial, and viral genes that cannot occur in nature or in traditional crossbreeding and could be unstable in the natural growing environment.

Organic food gardens can be as useful as they are beautiful. Whether they are messy or tidy, large or small, gardens are a place of refuge and health and can contribute greatly to your well-being. Gardens such as this one found at Chanticleer outside Philadelphia, Pennsylvania, can help feed the community and make a difference for you personally.

Continued from page 39

pests and foraging animals. Never use human, dog, or cat manure/feces as it can contain diseases and pathogens that can be harmful.

Your compost pile should be moist to the touch, like a wrung-out sponge, but not soaking wet. This moisture, plus the alternating layers, creates heat, microbial growth, and decomposition. Usually, it takes between three to four weeks to make compost, if the pile or composter is in full sun and you turn the materials regularly.

Examples of browns:
- Aged grass clippings
- Brown paper bags and shredded cardboard
- Newspaper; black-and-white soy print is best
- Shredded cotton and paper-based tissues and towels
- Straw
- Dead leaves from healthy plants (do not use diseased plants)

Examples of greens:
- Coffee grounds
- New grass clippings
- Tea bags with metal staple and string removed
- Pulled weeds and plant prunings (do not add prunings from diseased plants)
- Kitchen fruit and vegetable scraps. Avoid items that will root, such as potato skins and onions, unless ground completely

LEARN TO WATER CORRECTLY

Watering your plants correctly is absolutely critical for gardening success. Water too much and your plants drown; water too little and they dry up and die. No matter where you garden—high-rise balcony, suburban patio, or country farm—finding a way to get water to your plants is a critical concern.

If you have an organic garden, consider utilizing a drinking water–safe garden hose to water your plants. Traditional hoses are filled with chemicals. If you would not drink out of the hose, the water certainly should not be going on the vegetables, fruits, and herbs you might be consuming. Mulch your plants with natural materials such as compost, old leaves, or shredded bark to help hold moisture in the soil.

City water often contains fluoride and chlorine, which are not ideal nutrients choices for your plants. Collecting rainwater from rooftops prevents strain on storm water systems and enables you to water your plants without the chemicals found in city water. Rain barrels, cisterns, and other rain collection systems also help reduce the strain on residential water systems, whose use grows approximately 40 percent in hot summers because of outdoor landscape needs. Using a natural resource like rain barrel water also saves you money. Rain barrels need to be drained at the end of the gardening season, but outside of that, they are a fairly low-maintenance garden tool once installed.

Finally, your plant choices affect water use. If you can group plants with similar water and sunlight needs, your time spent watering and your water use will be reduced. Also water deeply once or twice per week when needed, rather than light or shallow watering every day.

FIND THE RIGHT LIGHT

Sunlight conditions vary, and understanding your sun conditions can make or break your garden's

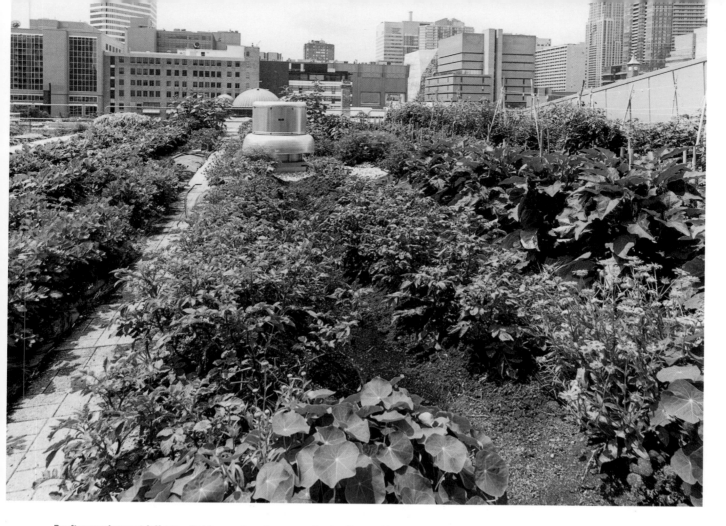

Rooftop gardens get full sun—but for most gardeners, understanding sunlight is a large concern. Study your light patterns closely and choose plantings that thrive in your unique sun conditions.

success. Carefully follow the directions on your seed packages or plant labels to make sure you have the right growing conditions. Full-sun plants need at least six hours of direct sunlight per day. Part-sun plants often prefer filtered light during the day but still need four hours of sunlight per day. Shade plants can live with little or no sunlight but still prefer indirect light to no light whatsoever. Of course, considering varying strength of

sun comes into place for potential gardening microclimates as well.

After the plants or seeds are in the ground and growing starts, watch your garden carefully to see if it needs water or organic amendments. Growing a garden, touching the soil with your hands, connecting with plants, and breathing in the fresh air can be the beginning of a wellness lifestyle that connects you to a mindful wellness journey.

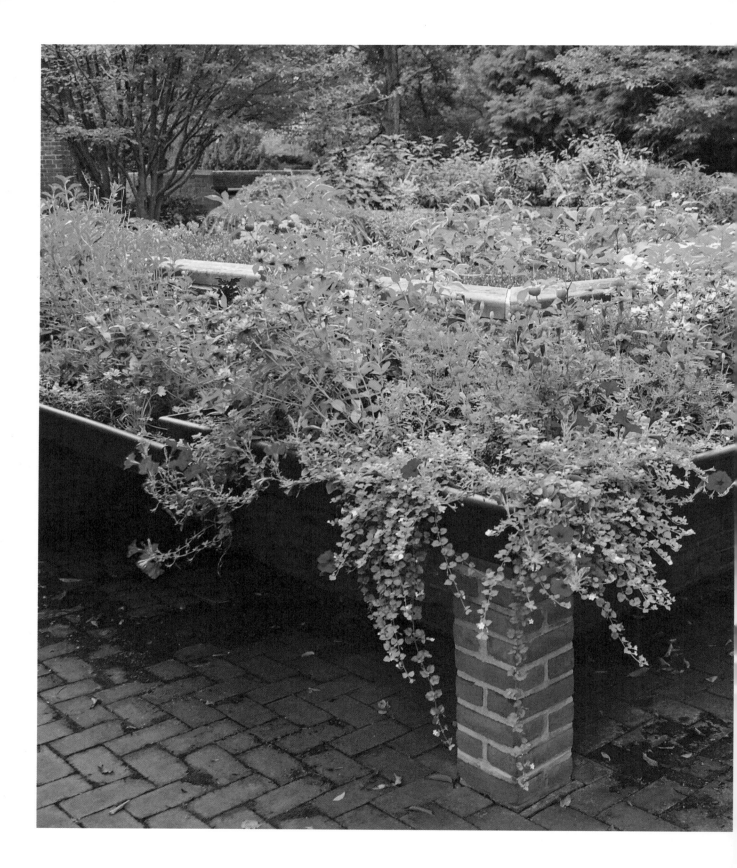

3

HEALTH-FRIENDLY ELEVATED BEDS, LIVING WALLS, AND CONTAINER GARDENS

ELEVATED BEDS

GROWING IN ELEVATED beds that are a meter (or more) high makes gardening much easier because it enables you to garden without bending over. Whether you have a condition like severe spinal degenerative osteoarthritis, like I do, or you just want an easier garden experience, elevated gardens are for you.

Elevated bed gardening also brings the sight and scent of flowers and herbs up closer to a person's eye and nose level. This can mean that it can also be used to enhance gardening for people who have reduced sight or smell abilities as well for those who do not. Emotionally therapeutic gardens often contain herbs and other scented plants that enhance anyone's mental well-being.

To plant an elevated bed, simply assemble your elevated system, then fill it with your preferred soil mix (more on appropriate soil mixes later in this chapter) up to a level about 2 inches or 5 centimeters from the top of the bed. This leaves room for watering.

Whether you start with seeds, seedlings, or plants, plan your design with the eventual full size of

OPPOSITE: Gardening in elevated beds built for easier access can be just as lovely as gardening right in the ground. This elevated garden is built at the Chicago Botanic Garden. It enables chair or wheelchair access so that someone who cannot stand to garden will still have access. *Photo taken at Chicago Botanic Garden.*

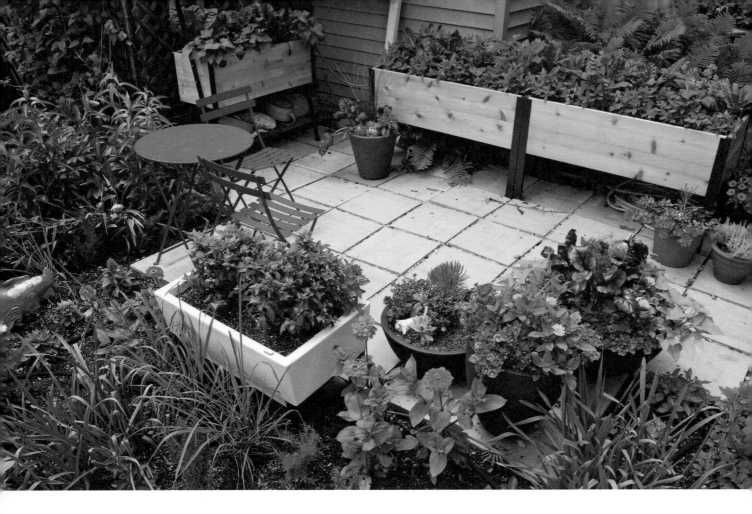

Building an elevated-bed patio garden can result in a beautiful, bountiful space that can be comfortably tended by a gardener who has a condition like osteoarthritis or rheumatoid arthritis. Additionally, such raised beds also lift plants up and away from pets and other garden pests. This lovely little patio garden is in front of the author's home within full view of her front walkway.

the plant in mind. If, for example, you plant a row of sweet potato vines with less than an inch between the plants, they will soon overcrowd one another. Follow planting directions on seed packets using the mature size of a plant as a spacing guide. Before you place vegetative plants, first arrange the plants on top of the soil. Once you have the proper spacing and design, dig a hole for each plant. Add a bit of organic fertilizer according to package directions, then gently bury each rootball, watering them in well.

If you have trouble digging, ask for help. I had my daughter assist with planting my elevated beds and have been grateful for the assistance.

LIVING WALLS

Container gardening with living wall systems makes it possible to produce large quantities of fruit, vegetables, herbs, tropicals, and flowers in a very small space. For instance, you could grow 40 plants in the same space as a window box simply by growing several levels of plants. In essence, a vertical garden or living wall is grown on the side of a fence, gate, building, or balcony. Most living wall systems have a structural support that is connected directly to a firm fence or wall, but they can also be stand-alone. Living wall units typically hold soil and plants, although some are hydroponic. Many systems have built-in watering tubes that can be directly connected to water lines.

One remarkable benefit of living wall gardening is, much like elevated beds, it raises plants up higher for easier access. From a wellness perspective, this is particularly important if a gardener has trouble bending or lifting. Living wall systems allow for easier access, plus they reduce common pest and disease problems because they offer increased air circulation and height: it can be challenging for a rabbit to climb a 6-foot fence to nibble on lettuce.

However, living walls do offer one important challenge: they hold less moisture than other traditional container gardens because of their positioning. When a living wall is raised a significant distance above the ground, it is more exposed to wind and air, which dries out the soil more quickly. A solution is to add a drip system to your living wall unit to keep watering regular. Increasing the weight and water-retention of your soil with additional organic ingredients can also help. (See *Water Retentive Container Garden Soil Mix Formula for Drought Conditions and Less Watering* in the Container Garden Soil Mix box

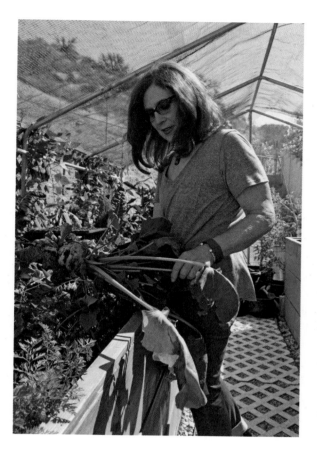

Jane Schwartz Gates, a writer and designer at Gates & Croft Horticultural Design, stands next to elevated vegetable beds in her Southern California greenhouse. She grows full-sized vegetables year round in the greenhouse, like the freshly harvested turnip she is holding. Jane says she enjoys food from the garden daily, so it helps her keep grocery costs down. The elevated beds make it easier on her back and joints to harvest and plant.

on page 51.) Great additions to your soil mix are worm castings and compost because both have the added benefit of adding more complexity to the soil, which will enhance microbial growth around the plants' root systems.

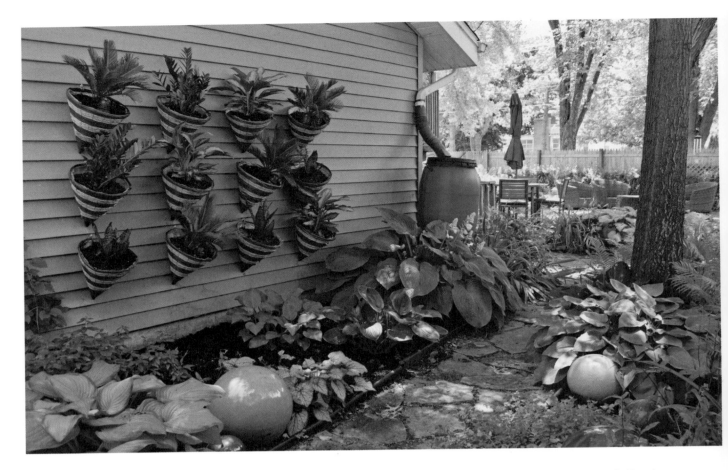

Planting a living wall with drought-tolerant houseplants, such the Plants of Steel line of plants from Costa Farms, can make it easier to maintain a garden wall because they require minimal attention and water. Plants featured in this garden are the ponytail palm, Chinese evergreen, sago palm, snake plant, and ZZ plant.

Growing living walls is easy—begin by building or purchasing a living wall system; hang according to directions in an area that has sufficient light for growing according to the plant requirements; use a water-retentive soil mix; use seeds, seedlings, or plants that are appropriate for the conditions that a wall garden presents; and water regularly. If you can plant your living wall garden with thriller, filler, and spiller design (see breakout box), your creation will be beautiful as well as be useful and therapeutic.

CONTAINER GARDENS

Traditional container gardens can be significantly smaller than a standard in-ground garden, but containers of all sorts can produce large quantities of food. While gardeners have always grown flowers in pots, producing organic herbs, vegetables, and fruit in garden containers is also easy.

For an edible plant to be organically grown in a container, one must consider the soil, the plants

Thriller, Filler, and Spiller Design Plan

Planting a container garden such as an elevated bed, living wall, or traditional pot with the thriller, filler, and spiller plan creates a full and eye-catching garden. You can mix different sorts of plants together, such as ornamental vegetables and herbs with traditional annual flowers, or you can create a centralized theme of all vegetable plants or all tropical plants. You just need to combine a thriller, a filler, and a spiller (ideally, with the same or similar water, soil, and sun requirements).

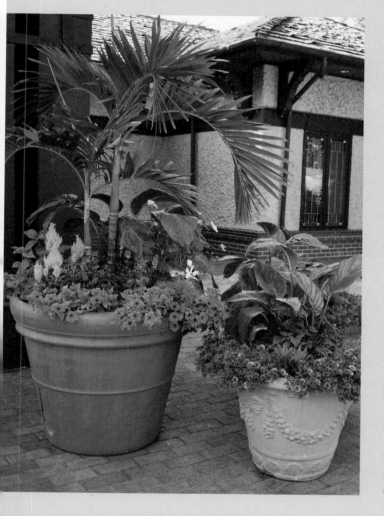

Thriller—Centerpiece plants that are bold, large, colorful, or architectural are known as thrillers. It will be your container superstar. In a living wall, one might plant the thriller toward the back of the wall, leaving room for the filler and spiller in front. In a round planting pot, one might plant the thriller either at the very center of the container or at the back. Thrillers are often considered foundational plants that anchor the rest of the design complements.

Filler—These are full plants that offer abundant foliage or flowers, but do not overpower the centerpiece thriller plant in size or color. In container gardens, fillers are plants that are positioned mostly in the middle, between the spiller and thriller. They are often plants that mound to surround the thriller. Fillers are essential in a container design in order to add rich color undertones, mass, and texture.

Spiller—Often spiller plants are known as *sprawlers*. They flow over and outside their container boundary. Spillers are most frequently vining plants or plants that spill out of the container and reach toward the ground. In a living wall, a spiller can effectively hide the planting unit. For elevated beds and container gardens, spillers break up the architecture of a planting container and soften its edges, adding an interesting place for the eye to trail around the composition of your planting design.

Thriller-filler-spiller container design is all about having a tall or boldly architectural feature plant in the center or back of a container, a fuller plant in the middle area of the containers, and a spilling plant at the edge of the planting. This design, found at Biltmore Estate in Asheville, North Carolina, is simple and easy to adopt for living walls, container gardens, and elevated beds even if you have very little design experience.

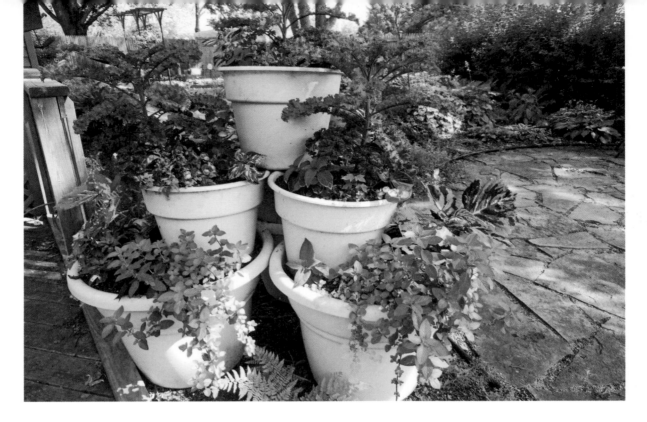

A stacked container garden, if securely placed for safety, can be a creative way to lift up a garden to a more accessible working height for someone who suffers chronic pain.

(either purchased or grown from organic seed), the contents of the water, and the container itself. Each pot must be safe and free of chemicals. Food-safe containers are made from glass, ceramic, stone, untreated wood, and food-safe plastics. Still concerned about the composition of a container, particularly if it is made of plastic or another manufactured material? Confirm by calling the company and asking direct questions about its manufacturing process.

Another idea for container gardening is to purchase a self-watering container in order to reduce the amount of watering regularly required. Container garden drip systems can also be installed to reduce the amount of maintenance required for your container gardens. Reduced maintenance means reduced strain on your joints and back by lessening the frequency or intensity required to maintain your gardens.

Once you have selected a container or planting system, do the same astute research with your soil. Use potting mix, manure compost, and worm castings that have been certified organic or make sure you know where the specific natural ingredients originated. During the planting process you might add fertilizer. Make sure the package speaks about the fertilizer being organic and safe to use in organic gardens.

Much like with elevated bed and living wall planting, planting up a container garden is fairly simple. Find a pot or container that works for your planting area; place the container where it will have sufficient light for growing; use a water-retentive soil mix; plant seeds, seedlings, or plants; and water regularly. Consider using the Thriller, Filler, and Spiller design plan (see breakout box), but feel free to break the rules and go outside of traditional design to find your own creative expression. Mix in lots of ornamental edible plants, scented plants, and colorful foliage.

An important rule with containers and wall gardens: they must have their soil replaced annually. Without the ability to bring new microbes and natural structure into the soil like you get when you plant in ground, the soil will be robbed of its nutrients by the plants annually. If you can't totally replace the soil, at least amend it with lots of rich, rotted material annually.

Whenever possible, grow plants from organic seed. When I cannot grow my plants from seed, I often struggle to find organic plants in the garden centers. Because of this, I follow a personal gardening policy of finding plants that are grown from seed in the most natural conditions possible. If the plants were not grown in organic conditions and I cannot find an organic substitute, I sometimes will still purchase a plant and grow it in my garden as organically as I can from the moment it touches the soil in my elevated beds and gardens. If, however, you are an organic purist or have severe medical restrictions and cannot produce your own seed, try connecting with friends in your community who can.

Water is another concern. According to the Ecology Center in Ann Arbor, Michigan, traditional garden hoses are made from

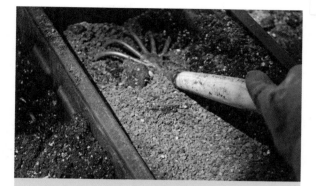

Using a custom container garden soil mix makes sense for your garden containers because it enables you to help your plants by meeting their individual soil needs. The right mix can mean significant water savings and a healthier root systems. Mix in organic fertilizer, following the directions on the fertilizer package for best results.

Container Garden Soil Mixes

Water-retentive container garden soil mix for dry conditions:
- ⅓ part organic potting soil with worm castings
- ⅓ part organic rotted composted manure
- ⅓ part plain compost

Standard container garden soil mix for general planting:
- ⅓ part organic potting soil with worm castings
- ⅓ part organic rotted composted manure or plain compost
- ⅓ part coarse builder's sand

Living wall soil mix formula:
- 1 part organic potting soil
- 1 part plain composted manure or plain compost
- 1 part pre-soaked coir peat
- 1 part vermiculite
- ⅛ part worm castings

Cactus and succulent soil mix:
- ⅓ part organic potting soil with worm castings
- ⅓ part perlite
- ⅓ part coarse builder's sand

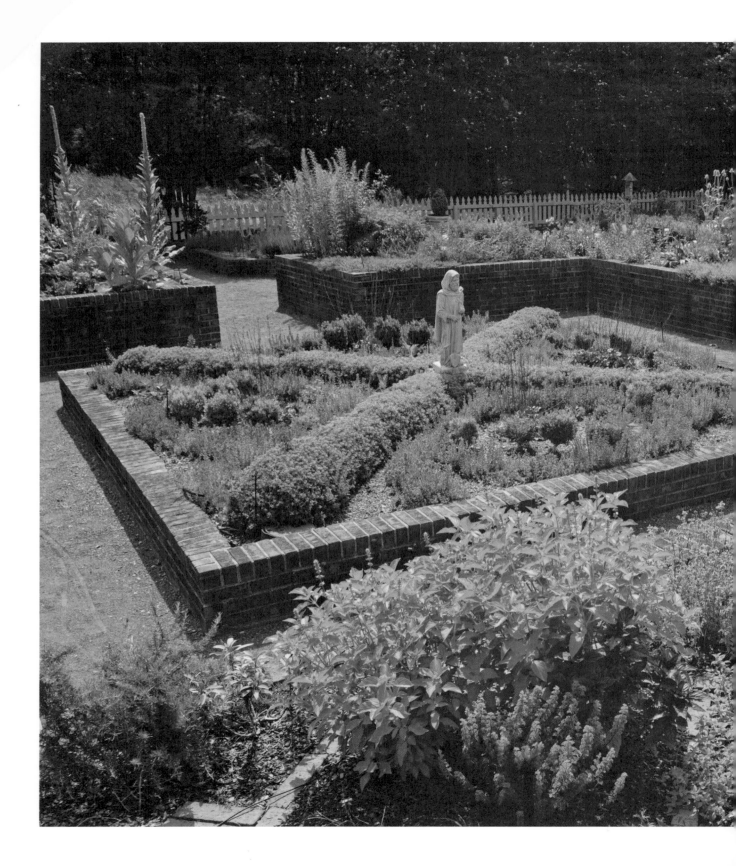

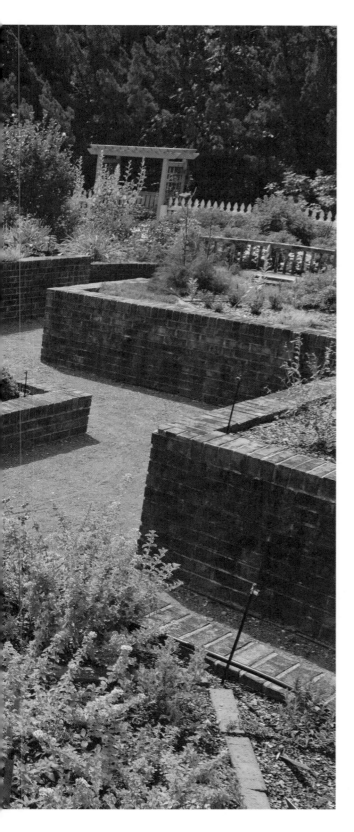

materials that are full of lead, bromine, and phthalates, toxic chemicals that are connected with learning impairments, birth defects, liver toxicity, and many other health issues. Watering your garden with a traditional garden hose might be providing your herbs, fruits, and vegetables with a heavy dose of unwanted chemicals. The Ecology Center recommends choosing hoses and drip systems labeled "drinking water-safe," specifically those made of polyurethane with lead-free fittings.

SPECIAL SOIL CONSIDERATIONS

Gardening in an elevated bed, living wall, or containers is different than gardening in ground, where the soil is rejuvenated by natural components that support plant health. Simply opening a bag of potting soil and tossing it into a pot does not ensure a successful container garden, nor will using soil dug straight from the ground. Creating a soil combination built for the specific plants growing in a container makes a better growing medium that will help you be successful as a container gardener.

One of my container garden secrets is to mix my favorite organic potting soil mix with amendments (see sidebar on page 51). Only add natural or organic ingredients into your container soil; do not mix in non-certified organic water polymers or crystals, artificial fertilizers, or other chemicals. Focus on your personal wellness by only using organic and natural ingredients.

This herb garden at the Huntsville Botanical Garden in Huntsville, Alabama, is a mix of elevated beds, raised beds, and containers, all of which make it easier to access.

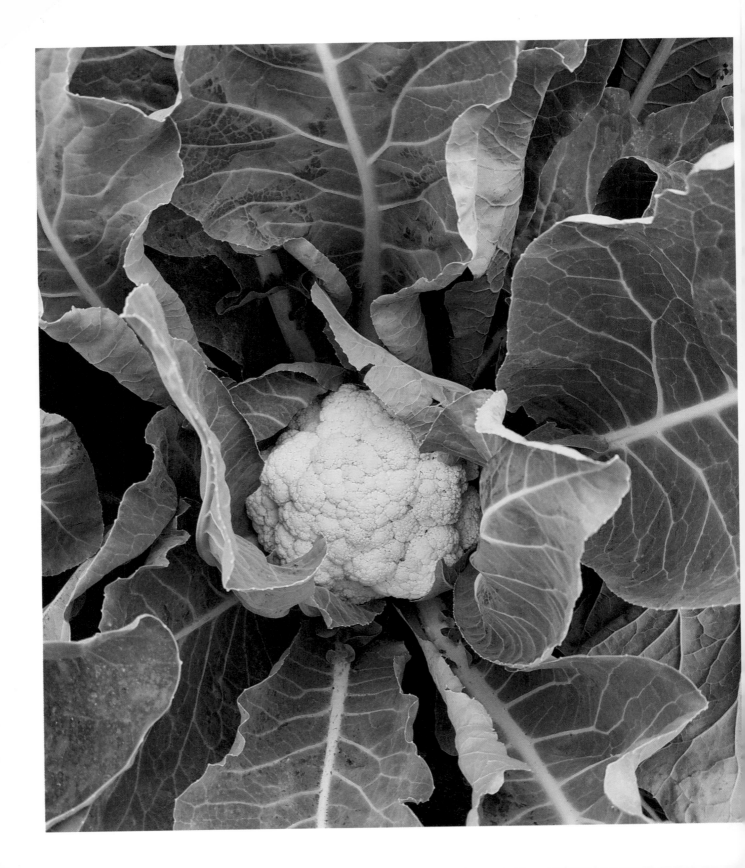

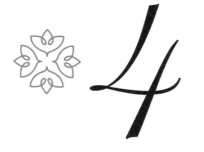

4

GROWING FOR NUTRITION
AND VITAMINS

WHEN I WAS a child, my father and I lived on a small street in a small town. An elderly lady watched me, and she also happened to rent our spare bedroom. She was a nanny for all intents and purposes, and she indulged me in all my little-girl plans and schemes. One such adventure was my very first gardening experience. We were sitting in the kitchen eating the most delicious cherries when I bit into a pit. That's when my babysitter told me that a tiny seed could grow into a giant tree. Fascinated, I begged her to allow me to plant the cherry seeds in the back garden. I put on my rain boots and went out in the mud to do the digging and burying, but alas, the tree never grew. Failure did not daunt me: I was infatuated with the soil and the seeds and the growing. I craved getting dirty by digging in the soil, and her indulging my play and curiosity triggered a lifetime addiction to soil, plants, and nature—but more importantly, it taught me a lesson that helped me connect nutrition to growing. The fruits and vegetables we eat come from the soil.

We can grow our own nutrition and health. Digging in the soil is a valuable step to wellness because of that magical bacterium strain,

OPPOSITE: Cauliflower, while low in fiber and other nutritive values, is extremely high in potassium with strong folate and vitamin C content as well. The leaves of cauliflower, such as this variety, called 'Minuteman', are often a beautiful blue-green, which makes the plant a beautiful and nutritious candidate for your garden.

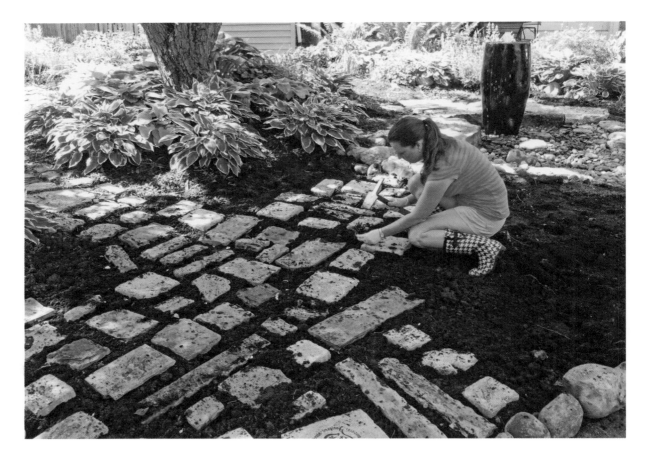

Digging in soil stirs up the bacterium strain, *Mycobacterium vaccae*, which stimulates release of serotonin in the brain and resulting in an instant mood boost. This healthful gardening byproduct is enhanced further when you grow your own organic herbs and vegetables because you are consuming the nutrients created within that soil.

Mycobacterium vaccae. Scientists believe that the bacteria found in soil stimulates serotonin, a chemical neurotransmitter that can affect mood, memory, sleep, sexual arousal, and social behavior. Serotonin boosts happen with direct skin-to-dirt contact and are remarkably important all through life. The most convenient place to find that effect is through gardening.

Growing your own food is important, too, in order to increase the level of nutritional value in the vegetables and fruits we consume. For instance, foods that are harvested fresh from the plant and immediately consumed are more likely to have a higher nutritive value. This value is critical for bodily function.

VITAMINS AND ANTIOXIDANTS

Fresh vegetables, fruits, and herbs have high levels of vitamins, minerals, and antioxidants, not to mention fiber. We cannot create these things within our bodies, so we have to find nutritious foods that will do more than simply satisfy our hunger but will also supply the critical items we need to stay healthy.

But what exactly are vitamins and antioxidants?

Vitamins

A vitamin is an organic compound that cannot be made by your body but which is necessary for proper health. So, we must regularly ingest vitamins. When you pick an absolutely delicious vegetable at the peak of freshness from your garden, you are getting the highest vitamin content possible, something that is often not possible at the supermarket. It can also be difficult to find a wide variety of fresh *organic* vegetables in your supermarket's produce section, fresh or not so fresh. Growing your own food solves these problems.

Which vitamin-rich plants should you grow organically in your garden? Use the vitamin guide (see pages 58–59, 61) and consult with your nutritionist and doctor. We know that green leafy and cruciferous vegetables have performed particularly well in disease prevention studies. However, based on your health tests and medical professional's recommendations, you might grow foods that specifically fit your personal health history requirements. For instance, if you are low in vitamin A, you might try swiss chard, sweet potato, parsley, carrots, basil, kale, lettuce, bok choy, or spinach.

Outside of specific recommendations from your medical professionals, consider which herbs, fruits, and vegetables you like and which might have higher nutritional content. Also spend time experimenting with unusual vegetables that might not be commonly found at the grocer, but can bring variety, taste, and color to your plate like chayote squash, beets, endive, or fennel.

If you do not have your handy-dandy vitamin guide with you when thinking about seed or plant purchases for gardening, one rule to remember is that the more color a vegetable has, the more vitamins and nutrients it is likely to have. One of my favorite ornamental edible container design combinations is swiss chard, kale, arugula, and parsley. All have remarkably bold color and interesting leaf design. They also happen to be filled with lots of vitamins and fiber.

Growing vitamin-filled food is good for you, but consider this: whatever you cannot consume immediately can be frozen, canned, or donated to your local food pantry. From an overall wellness standpoint, sharing your bounty with your friends, family, and neighbors is good for everyone. That brings wellness to your body and your mind.

ANTIOXIDANTS

Antioxidants are substances that can constrain oxidation, a process that can cause cell damage in your body. Each human body creates oxidants to defend against invading viruses and microbes—that's good. But you can also encounter negative oxidants in the environment as well, such as air pollution, alcohol, cigarette smoke, and chemical exposure. If you have too many oxidants they can cause cell damage and lead to chronic health issues such as Alzheimer's, vision loss, cancer, and heart disease. Consuming antioxidants is nutritionally good for your body.

Home-Grown Fruits and Vegetables Nutrition

Most whole vegetables and fruits that home gardeners can grow in their home gardens are fairly low in glycemic value, with only a few exceptions. Review this chart for lower glycemic index, high fiber, and high vitamin foods you might be able to grow yourself.

Fruits and Vegetables	Serving Size (g)	Glycemic Index	Calories (kcal)	Protein (g)	Carbohydrate (g)	Fiber (g)	Calcium (mg)	Iron (mg)	Phosphorus (mg)	Potassium (mg)	Vitamin C (mg)	Vitamin A (IU)	Vitamin E (mg)
Apple	120	36.2	62	0.31	16.57	2.9	7	0.14	13	128	5.5	65	0.22
Apricot	120	45.5	58	1.68	13.34	2.4	16	0.47	28	311	12	2,311	1.07
Arugula	100	32	25	2.58	3.65	1.6	160	1.46	52	369	15	2,373	0.43
Artichoke	100	32	47	3.27	10.51	5.4	44	1.28	90	370	11.7	13	0.19
Asparagus	100	32	20	2.2	3.88	2.1	24	2.14	52	202	5.6	756	1.13
Avocado	100	50	160	2	8.53	6.7	12	0.55	52	485	10	146	2.07
Banana	120	53.3	107	1.31	27.41	3.1	6	0.31	26	430	10.4	77	0.12
Banana Pepper	100	32	27	1.66	5.35	3.4	14	0.46	32	256	82.7	340	0.69
Basil	100	N/A	23	3.15	2.65	1.6	177	3.17	56	295	18	5,275	0.8
Beets	100	64	43	1.61	9.56	2.8	16	0.8	40	325	4.9	33	0.04
Bitter Melon	100	32	17	1	3.7	2.8	19	0.43	31	296	84	471	0
Blackberries	100	N/A	43	1.39	9.61	5.3	29	0.62	22	162	21	214	1.17
Blueberries	100	40	57	0.74	14.49	2.4	6	0.28	12	77	9.7	54	0.57
Bok Choy	100	N/A	13	1.5	2.18	1	105	0.8	37	252	45	4,468	0.09
Broccoli	100	32	34	2.82	6.64	2.6	47	0.73	66	316	89.2	623	0.78
Brussels Sprouts	100	32	43	3.38	8.95	3.8	42	1.4	69	389	85	754	0.88
Cabbage, Green	100	32	25	1.28	5.8	2.5	40	0.47	26	170	36.6	98	0.15
Cantaloupe	120	67.5	41	1.01	9.79	1.1	11	0.25	18	320	44	4,058	0.06
Carrots	80	16	33	0.74	7.66	2.2	26	0.24	28	256	4.7	13,365	0.53
Cassava	100	46	160	1.36	38.06	1.8	16	0.27	27	271	20.6	13	0.19
Cauliflower	100	32	25	1.92	4.97	2	22	0.42	44	299	48.2	0	0.08
Celeriac	100	N/A	42	1.5	9.2	1.8	43	0.7	115	300	8	0	0.36
Celery	100	32	16	0.69	2.97	1.6	40	0.2	24	260	3.1	449	0.27
Chard, Swiss	100	32	19	1.8	3.74	1.6	51	1.8	46	379	30	6,116	1.89
Chayote	100	N/A	19	0.82	4.51	1.7	17	0.34	18	125	7.7	0	0.12
Cherry	120	22	76	1.27	19.21	2.5	16	0.43	25	266	8.4	77	0.08
Cilantro	100	32	23	2.13	3.67	2.8	67	1.77	48	521	27	6,748	2.5
Corn	115	58	99	3.76	21.5	2.3	2	0.6	102	310	7.8	215	0.08
Cucumber	100	32	12	0.59	2.16	0.7	14	0.22	21	136	3.2	72	0.03
Dates	60	45.2	166	1.09	44.98	4	38	0.54	37	418	0	89	0
Eggplant	100	32	25	0.98	5.88	3	9	0.23	24	229	2.2	23	0.03
Endive	100	32	17	1.25	3.35	3.1	52	0.83	28	314	6.5	2,167	0.44
Fennel, Bulb	100	N/A	31	1.24	7.3	3.1	49	0.73	50	414	12	963	0.58
Fennel Seeds	50	N/A	172	7.9	26.14	19.9	598	9.27	244	847	10.5	68	0
Figs	100	61	74	0.75	19.18	2.9	35	0.37	14	232	2	142	0.11

Sources: www.diabetes.org/food-and-fitness/food/what-can-i-eat/understanding-carbohydrates/glycemic-index-and-diabetes.html, www.dietgrail.com/gid, www.glycemicindex.com/foodSearch.php, ndb.nal.usda.gov/ndb/search/list, www.nutritionsoftware.org/usda-nutrient-databases

Fruits and Vegetables	Serving Size (g)	Glycemic Index	Calories (kcal)	Protein (g)	Carbohydrate (g)	Fiber (g)	Calcium (mg)	Iron (mg)	Phosphorus (mg)	Potassium (mg)	Vitamin C (mg)	Vitamin A (IU)	Vitamin E (mg)
Garlic	100	32	149	6.36	33.06	2.1	181	1.7	153	401	31.2	9	0.08
Grapefruit	120	25	38	0.76	9.7	1.3	14	0.11	10	167	41.3	1,112	0.16
Grapes	120	46	80	0.76	20.58	1.1	17	0.35	12	229	4.8	120	0.23
Honeydew Melon	100	65	36	0.54	9.09	0.8	6	0.17	11	228	18	50	0.02
Jicama	100	32	38	0.72	8.82	4.9	12	0.6	18	150	20.2	21	0.46
Kale	100	32	49	4.28	8.75	3.6	150	1.47	92	491	120	9,990	1.54
Kiwi	120	52.5	73	1.37	17.59	3.6	41	0.37	41	374	111.2	104	1.75
Lettuce, Romaine	100	32	17	1.23	3.29	2.1	33	0.97	30	247	4	8,710	0.13
Leeks	100	N/A	61	1.5	14.15	1.8	59	2.1	35	180	12	1,667	0.92
Lemon	100	N/A	29	1.1	9.32	2.8	26	0.6	16	138	53	22	0.15
Lime	100	N/A	30	0.7	10.54	2.8	33	0.6	18	102	29.1	50	0.22
Lychee	100	57	66	0.83	16.53	1.3	5	0.31	31	171	71.5	0	0.07
Mango	120	51	72	0.98	17.98	1.9	13	0.19	17	202	43.7	1,298	1.08
Mushrooms	100	32	22	3.09	3.26	1	3	0.5	86	318	2.1	0	0.01
Okra	100	32	33	1.93	7.45	3.2	82	0.62	61	299	23	716	0.27
Onions	100	32	40	1.1	9.34	1.7	23	0.21	29	146	7.4	2	0.02
Orange	120	42	56	1.13	14.1	2.9	48	0.12	17	217	63.8	270	0.22
Papaya	120	59	52	0.56	12.98	2	24	0.3	12	218	73.1	1,140	0.36
Parsley	100	32	36	2.97	6.33	3.3	138	6.2	58	554	133	8,424	0.75
Parsnips	80	52	57	1.06	13.61	2.9	30	0.46	55	294	10.4	0	0.8
Peach	120	42	47	1.09	11.45	1.8	7	0.3	24	228	7.9	391	0.88
Peas	100	48	81	5.42	14.45	5.7	25	1.47	108	244	40	765	0.13
Pears	100	38	57	0.36	15.23	3.1	9	0.18	12	116	4.3	25	0.12
Pineapple	120	66	54	0.66	14.18	0	16	0.3	11	150	20.3	62	0
Potatoes	150	85	116	3.07	26.23	3.2	18	1.22	86	638	29.5	3	0.01
Prunes	60	29	144	1.31	38.33	4.3	26	0.56	41	439	0.4	469	0.26
Pumpkin	100	75	26	1	6.5	0.5	21	0.8	44	340	9	8,513	1.06
Radishes	100	32	16	0.68	3.4	1.6	25	0.34	20	233	14.8	7	0
Raisins	60	65	179	1.84	47.51	2.2	30	1.13	61	449	1.4	0	0.07
Raspberries	100	N/A	52	1.2	11.94	6.5	25	0.69	29	151	26.2	33	0.87
Rhubarb	100	N/A	21	0.9	4.54	1.8	86	0.22	14	288	8	102	0.27
Rutabaga	150	72	56	1.62	12.93	3.4	64	0.66	80	458	37.5	3	0.45
Serrano Pepper	100	32	32	1.74	6.7	3.7	11	0.86	40	305	44.9	937	0.69
Shallots	100	N/A	72	2.5	16.8	3.2	37	1.2	60	334	8	4	0.04
Spinach	100	32	23	2.86	3.63	2.2	99	2.71	49	558	28.1	9,377	2.03
Strawberries	100	N/A	32	0.67	7.68	2	16	0.41	24	153	58.8	12	0.29
Summer Squash	100	32	17	1.21	3.11	1	16	0.37	38	261	17.9	200	0.12
Sweet Pepper, Red	100	32	31	0.99	6.03	2.1	7	0.43	26	211	127.7	3,131	1.58
Sweet Potato	150	77	129	2.35	30.18	4.5	45	0.92	70	506	3.6	21,280	0.39
Tomatoes	100	38	18	0.88	3.89	1.2	10	0.27	24	237	13.7	833	0.54
Turnip	100	62	28	0.9	6.43	1.8	30	0.3	27	191	21	0	0.03
Watermelon	120	76	36	0.73	9.06	0.5	8	0.29	13	134	9.7	683	0.06
Zucchini	100	N/A	21	2.71	3.11	1.1	21	0.79	93	459	34.1	490	0

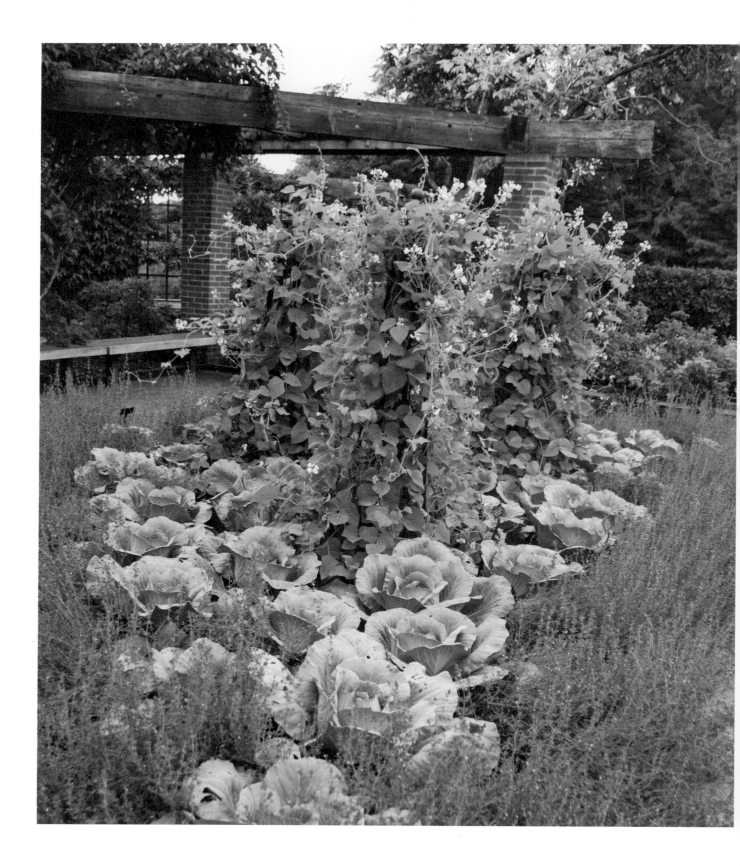

Home-grown Nutrition

Beans have high fiber, potassium, and protein content. This chart shows a breakout of the glycemic index as well as the vitamin, fiber, and protein content for different varieties of beans.

Beans/Legumes/ Lentils	Serving Size (g)	Glycemic Index	Calories (kcal)	Protein (g)	Carbohydrate (g)	Fiber (g)	Calcium (mg)	Iron (mg)	Phosphorus (mg)	Potassium (mg)	Vitamin C (mg)	Vitamin A (IU)	Vitamin E (mg)
Black Beans	150	30	512	32.4	93.54	23.2	184	7.53	5.28	2,224	0	26	0.32
Black Soy Beans	100	16	446	36.49	30.16	9.3	277	15.7	704	1,797	6	22	0.85
Black-Eyed Peas	150	50	504	35.28	90.05	15.9	165	12.4	636	1,668	2.2	75	0.58
Cannellini Beans	150	31	116	8.07	23.07	6.9	69	1.67	0	312	0	0	0
Edamame	100	N/A	109	11.22	7.61	4.8	60	2.11	161	482	9.7	0	0.72
Fava Beans	100	N/A	341	26.12	58.29	25	103	6.7	421	1,062	1.4	53	0.05
Garbanzo Beans	150	32	567	30.7	94.43	18.3	86	6.46	378	1,077	6	100	1.23
Green Lentils	150	30	540	39	90	45	60	10.8	0	0	7.2	0	0
Kidney Beans	150	34	500	35.37	90.02	37.3	214	12.3	610	2,109	6.8	0	0.33
Lima Beans	150	32	507	32.19	95.07	28.5	122	11.27	578	2,586	0	0	1.08
Mung Beans	150	36.5	520	35.79	93.93	24.5	198	10.11	550	1,869	7.2	171	0.77
Navy Beans	150	39	506	33.49	90.12	23	220	8.23	610	1,778	0	0	0.03
Northern Beans	100	N/A	339	21.86	62.37	20.2	175	5.47	447	1,387	5.3	0	0.22
Pinto Beans	150	36	520	32.13	93.82	23.2	170	7.61	616	2,090	9.4	0	0.32
Red Lentils	150	24.6	537	35.87	94.65	16.2	72	11.08	441	1,002	2.5	87	0
Yellow Lentils	150	28	528	36.95	95.03	16	52	9.77	422	1,016	6.8	58	0.73
White Beans	150	14	500	35.04	90.41	22.8	360	15.66	452	2,692	0	0	0.32

Sources: www.diabetes.org/food-and-fitness/food/what-can-i-eat/understanding-carbohydrates/glycemic-index-and-diabetes.html, www.dietgrail.com/gid, www.glycemicindex.com/foodSearch.php, ndb.nal.usda.gov/ndb/search/list, www.nutritionsoftware.org/usda-nutrient-databases

THE STRESS EFFECT

One of the reasons to increase nutritionally sound, vitamin-rich, and antioxidant-filled foods in our diets is that it can reduce stress. Eating a diet that is high in protein, vegetable, and fiber is low in sugars and fat, and it can reduce inflammation. Certain types of chronic pain and medical conditions depend on reduction of inflammation for improvement.

PLANT-BASED FOODS PROVIDE A BETTER LIFE

Selecting the herbs, fruits, and vegetables to grow in your garden that have the strongest nutritional values can enhance your wellness-centered diet. But one thing most doctors seem to agree on is that there is no single fruit, herb, seed, or vegetable that can provide *all* the nutrients you

OPPOSITE: Nutritional foods can be grown in an attractive fashion. These pea towers are surrounded by cabbage and thyme, creating a nutritious and artful scent-filled display. *Photo taken at Chicago Botanic Garden.*

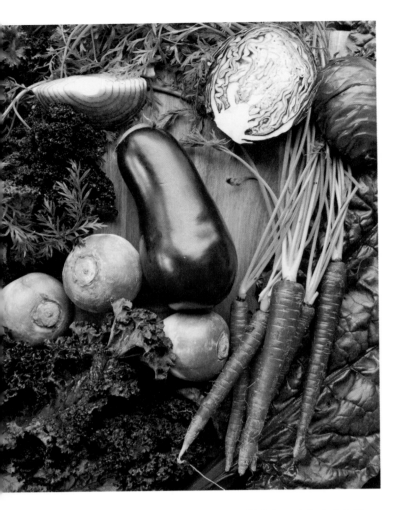

All fruits and vegetables are very likely to contribute to better health, but colorful vegetables and cruciferous vegetables are stronger champions for a preventative diet. This delicious purple selection of vegetables—onions, cabbage, carrots, eggplant, turnips, kale, and swiss chard—are full of nutritious benefits.

need to be healthy and well. Instead, the secret is to consume a diet filled with a variety of plant-based foods to help prevent cancer, heart disease, and stroke.

When I began my experimental diet and exercise routine with no grains, no dairy, and no sugar, plus walking daily, I felt it would not help me. I debated with my nutritionist and did my best to cheat on the diet, believing that food was not the cure for me. Truly, I was dooming myself to failure with that mindset. My certified nutritionist, Deepa Deshmukh, MPH, RD, BC-ADM, CDE, firmly insisted that I stay on my elimination diet for 30 days without cheating. She felt that while not everyone with chronic pain has inflammation, chronic inflammation is significantly present during most chronic pain episodes and that I would find relief for my severe degenerative spinal osteoarthritis. As always, her mantra was, "Food is the cure!"

Her approach of eliminating allergens and potential trigger foods, reducing sugars including excessively sweet fruits and juices, while increasing my consumption of healthy fats, herbs, and vegetables had a surprising effect. Within a week I had close to 40 percent reduction in my chronic pain levels. Her prescribed diet, which contained a lot of fish and chicken combined with plant-based foods, helped reduce my problems. By the end of the 30 days, I was finally sleeping after six weeks of painful insomnia and living better after months of pain-filled movement. No one was more surprised than I was to discover the power of eating healthier.

A Harvard-based Nurses' Health Study and Health Professionals Follow-up Study is the longest modern study on dietary habits. The eating habits of approximately 110,000 women and men were followed for 14 years. Those participants who averaged more than eight

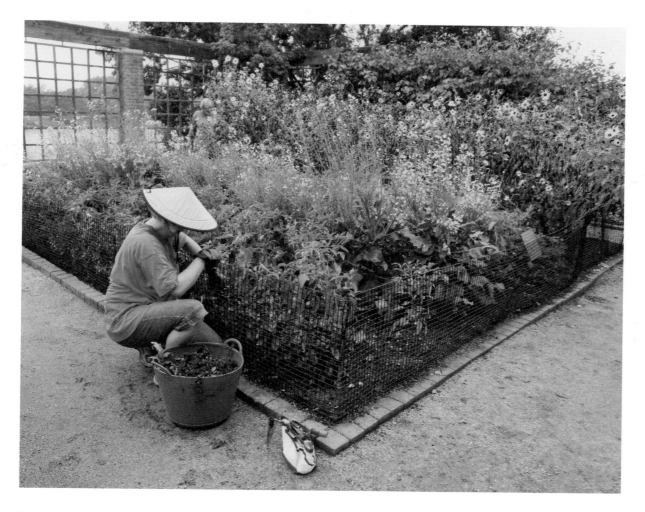

Colorful and flavorful vegetables sound delicious to you, but also to rabbits and other varmints. Elevating vegetable beds or putting a rabbit fence around your vegetable garden can assist you in keeping unwanted creatures away from your nutritious food. *Photo taken at Chicago Botanic Garden.*

servings of fruits and vegetables daily were at least 30 percent less likely to have a stroke or heart attack. According to the Harvard School of Public Health, "Although all fruits and vegetables likely contribute to this benefit, green leafy vegetables such as lettuce, spinach, swiss chard, and mustard greens; cruciferous vegetables such as broccoli, cauliflower, cabbage, Brussels sprouts, bok choy, and kale" all make important contributions to a stronger preventative diet.

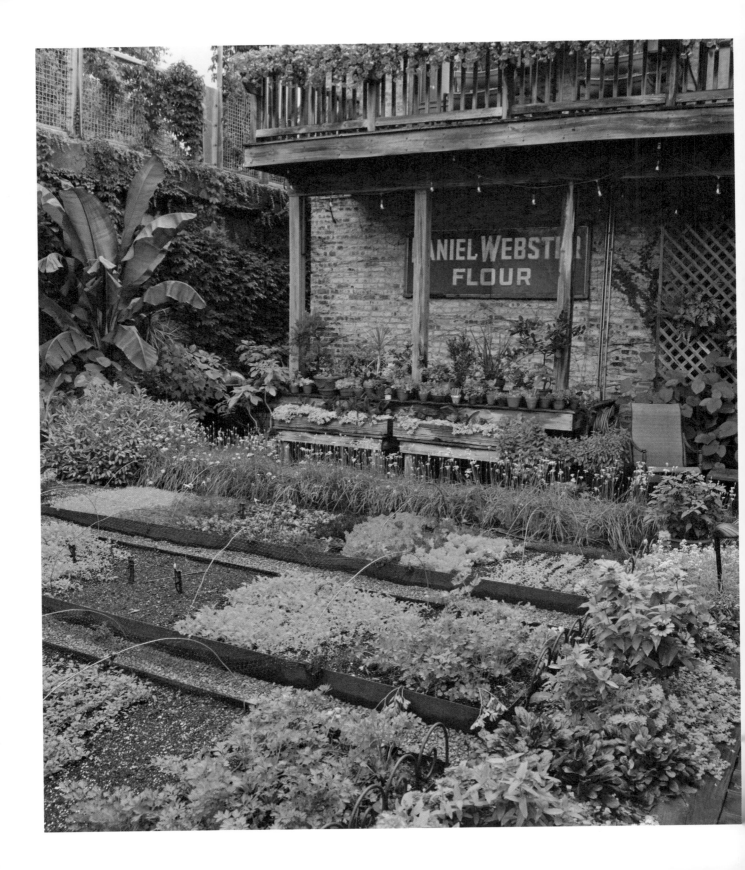

5

KITCHEN GARDEN INSPIRATION

A KITCHEN OR POTAGER garden is a special place. It is a garden where herbs, vegetables, and fruits are grown for use in cooking and eating. Growing your own food and using it as the center of your wellness program makes a lot of sense because you will also benefit from exercise, fresh air and sunshine, therapeutic scents, direct contact with soil, and organic foods. While a traditional potager is grown in the ground, you could also create your own organic garden in elevated beds, living walls, and container pots.

I want to start this chapter with a truly inspirational kitchen garden, which focuses very strongly on the phytonutrient-rich microgreens as its primary vegetable byproduct. Your garden will likely never grow to this size, but there are plenty of inspirational lessons to be learned here.

OPPOSITE: Chef Rick Bayless's inspiring and beautiful kitchen garden in Chicago's Bucktown neighborhood is filled with healthy microgreens, tomatoes, squash, and many ingredients you can find at his restaurants.

THE BAYLESS KITCHEN GARDENS

On a rainy summer day, I met Rick Bayless, award-winning cookbook author, television chef, famous restaurateur, and prolific philanthropist, in his very special kitchen garden in Chicago's Bucktown neighborhood. We talked about the benefits of growing your own fresh food and the importance of connecting food to wellness.

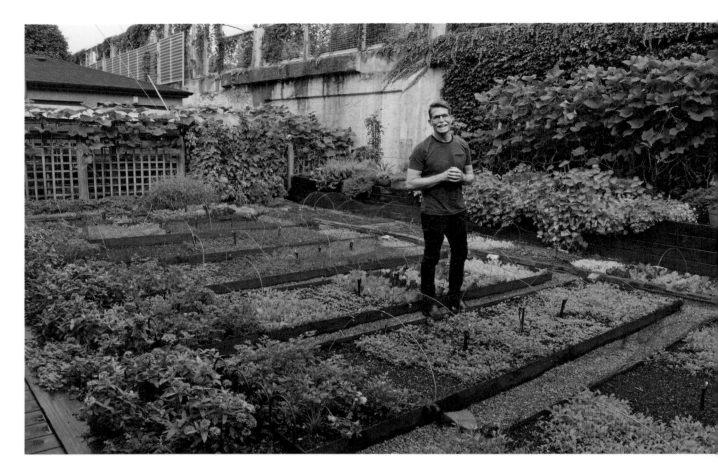

Rick Bayless stands in his garden in Chicago. In this 1,000-square-foot area of his backyard, Rick and his team produce 700 pounds of salad greens, 65,000 edible flowers, 250 pounds of herbs, and 100 pounds of butternut squash annually. Feeding people with healthy, wholesome, fresh food is what Rick claims is the solution for our fast-paced world—good food invites wellness because it makes us slow down to appreciate it.

Rick Bayless is full of passion when it comes to bringing food grown in healthy soil directly to the kitchen table and the health benefits it creates. When you meet Rick, you are struck with the fact that he lives the healthy life he evangelizes, that eating wholesome food and staying active can be a panacea for a stressfully busy life. While Rick spends the majority of his time running his restaurant empire and working on television, he works closely with a team that plants and manages his potager gardens. His delightfully jam-packed kitchen garden has a mix of in-ground, elevated, and container plantings that are in production for eight months of the year. In the 1,000-square-foot area of his backyard, he produces 700 pounds of salad greens, 65,000 edible flowers, 250 pounds of herbs, and 100 pounds of butternut squash annually.

Describing himself as endlessly curious, Rick says, "Understanding the intricacies of a potager garden is important to building a varied and healthy plate filled with authentic, real food." This starts at the level of soil and compost but extends all the way to harvest. When creating his PBS television series, "Mexico: One Plate at a Time," Rick explores authentic Mexican food and gets to see how food gardens and restaurants from many different states in Mexico use vegetables and herbs. He brings those ideas back to his own gardens and installs new plant varieties with the ongoing goal of growing locally and using non-processed garden fresh produce for his restaurants.

Mexican cuisine typically contains less meat but is high in beans, rice, and vegetables. "I have had many people tell me that tacos are fattening, yet eating tacos al pastor, for example, is significantly better for you because it is lower in fat and lower in sugar than consuming an energy bar. I use pork shoulder, chipotle chile en adobo sauce, achiote paste, onions, and pineapple in my recipe, then I serve it on a warm corn tortilla with tomatillo salsa. This is good food—real food—and it is so much better for you than eating a bar filled with ingredients that are not fresh."

Rick has learned from his hundreds of visits to the Mexican states that, "Mexicans often see meal time as an important break in their day that must be celebrated with friends and family. They perceive it as a 'sacred time to nourish myself' and growing your own fresh, natural, and hyper-local produce to contribute to that sacred meal is an important component of wellness and health." This is great inspiration for your own kitchen garden; growing your own food and consuming it in a thoughtful way encourages your body and mind to be well.

While your wellness potager garden might be much smaller than Rick's, it is possible to easily emulate his ideas. Be ever-curious, search out new ideas, and plant new varieties so that you can also grow nutrient-filled produce for your own family. Rick lives the wellness lifestyle by exploring nutrient values of various produce, experimenting with ethnic and regional cuisine, growing and buying local so his foods are fresher and more nutritious, and using the garden as a place of beauty as much as a place to produce the practical ingredients used in cooking meals.

RICK'S MICROGREENS

Microgreens take the front stage in Rick Bayless's garden. According to the US Department of Agriculture, microgreens are filled with concentrated levels of nutrients. Because of their bold colors and intense flavors, they are an excellent choice as a salad, in soups, on sandwiches, or as a beautiful garnish. Beneficially, they can be grown in less than a few weeks, which makes it possible to have multiple plantings and harvests per season.

According to Rick, growing microgreens, sometimes known as "vegetable confetti," is easy.

- Start seeds in a sunny window, container garden, or directly in the ground with at least four hours of light per day
- Follow seed packet directions
- Scatter seeds evenly on top of the soil, making sure the seeds are pressed down firmly
- Cover with a thin layer of soil
- Mist the soil and keep evenly moist
- Harvest in 6 to 21 days by trimming with scissors

Rick's microgreen-filled kitchen garden is the brainchild collaboration between he, Bill Shores, and Deann Bayless, who is the producer of Rick's PBS television series, founding partner of the Bayless restaurants, and his wife of more than 37 years. Bill Shores runs Urban Edible and is a Chicago-based grower who specializes in small-space-intensive food production and is the primary manager of the garden with his Urban Edible team. Their nutrient-rich microgreens are typically harvested and rushed to their restaurants then replanted in the very same day.

GROWING IN SHADE OR PART SHADE

Knowing that vegetables, fruits, and herbs prefer full sun, many gardeners, particularly those who live in urban environments like Rick Bayless, feel stymied when they consider establishing a

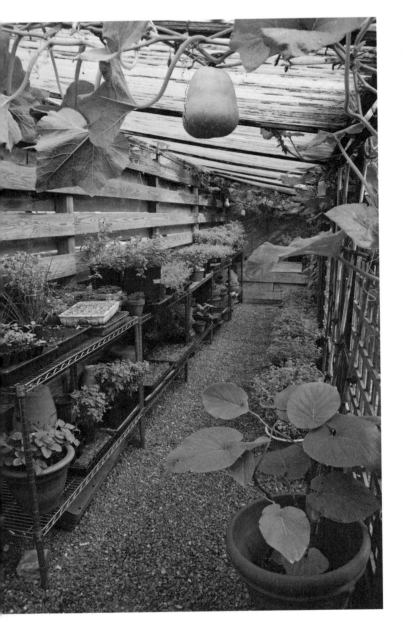

While Rick Bayless's microgreen garden is mostly direct seeded, the brain-child behind the garden's maintenance, Bill Shores and the team at Urban Edible, have a small plant potting area and seed-starting nursery at the back of Rick's property to help with any plant replacements needed throughout the season.

Shade-Tolerant Herbs and Vegetables

Growing vegetables and herbs on a part-shade balcony, patio, or traditional in-ground kitchen garden is possible. Part shade is defined as approximately two to four hours of sun per day. Leafy herbs and vegetables perform better in shadier conditions, while fruiting and rooting plants do not do as well.

- Arugula
- Basil
- Beans
- Beet greens
- Celery
- Collards
- Corn mache
- Endive
- Kale
- Lettuces
- Leafy herbs
- Malabar spinach
- Mustard greens
- Bok choy
- Peas
- Radishes
- Rhubarb
- Spinach
- Swiss chard
- Turnip greens

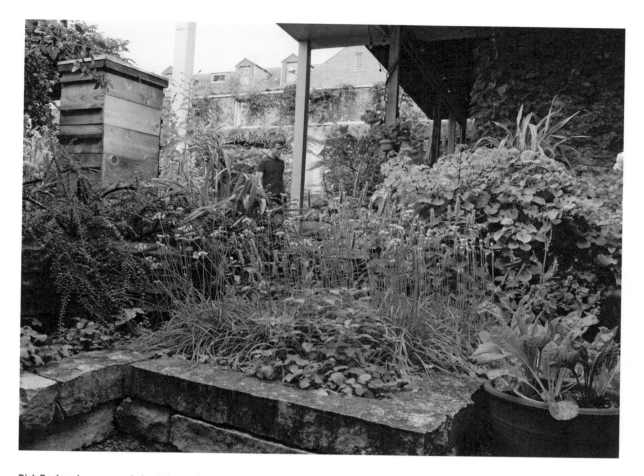

Rick Bayless is concerned about the environment and especially about the bee crisis in the United States. His beehive is part of his garden: the bees do a remarkable job of pollinating vegetables and herbs while simultaneously bringing honey to the kitchen garden.

kitchen garden. Although it might be more of a challenge to grow in the shade, it is surprisingly easy once you get started. Growing produce in shade opens up growing areas you might not have previously considered: on balconies, along fence lines, lining patios and walkways, and between buildings.

Living walls are particularly effective for a shade kitchen garden because they require less space. Produce such as leafy greens sometimes remain smaller when grown in heavy shade, so planting more closely together works well: you get smaller but more frequent harvests.

There is a rule to remember when planting in shade: no sun = no fruits and no roots. In other words, plants such as potatoes, which are roots, and tomatoes, which are fruits, are less likely to produce an abundant (or any) harvest in heavier

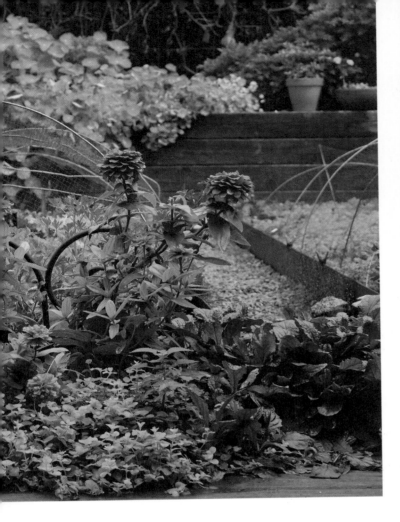

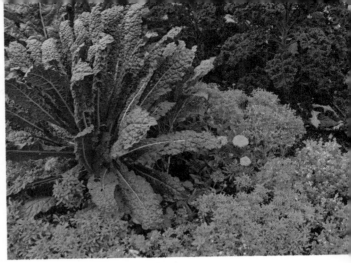

ABOVE: Kale is colorful, filled with nutritional value, and grows wonderfully in both sun and part-shade. Many leafy greens and herbs make great part-shade plants and work very well when tucked in between larger plants that shade out their partners as well. Utilizing leafy herbs and vegetables that have a variety of hues can brighten dark corners with happy color.

LEFT: One of the amazing things about an organic kitchen garden like Rick Bayless's Chicago plot is that it is useful, but also beautiful. Having a lovely garden filled with flowers attracts pollinators; this helps produce more vegetables, which in turn helps your family eat better. Spending time in your garden reduces stress and increases wellness, while eating the fruits of your labors guarantees a connection to improved nutrition.

shade. A convenient list of shade-tolerant herbs and vegetables that can grow well in a potager garden are listed in the sidebar on page 68.

THE HEAT- AND DROUGHT-TOLERANT KITCHEN GARDEN

With climate change and global warming, many areas of the world are experiencing unexpected heat and drought. It is also possible to have hotter microclimates in metropolitan areas where the "urban heat island effect" takes place. This is a phenomenon where air temperatures are higher due to the excessive amount of heat-retaining concrete, asphalt, and buildings that have replaced vegetation. Generally speaking, vegetation helps cool down the air at night, where the urban heat island effect keeps temperatures warmer at night, increasing overall temperatures more consistently.

With this added heat, gardeners are discovering that the soil in their planters and in ground sometimes require more water. If you live in a desert area or an area plagued with the urban heat island effect, why not plant your

CHAPTER 5

potager garden with heat and drought in mind by using drought-tolerant plants and vegetables?

You can conserve water in drought- or heat-affected gardens simply by reducing evaporation. Mulching in-ground, elevated, and container gardens can help keep soil moist longer. Utilizing worm castings and other natural soil amendments that are moisture-retentive can help. Planting in part-sun keeps the sun from burning plants and soil. Using drip irrigation systems and watering evenly and regularly also keep the soil moist.

Whether you live in a hot spot or not, planting drought-tolerant herbs and vegetables can mean less watering maintenance for you (see below). Conserving water saves time and money, which makes it easier to grow and maintain a kitchen potager garden.

Herbs and Vegetables for a Hot Dry Garden

Growing vegetables and herbs in your kitchen garden while living in a heat- or drought-plagued area is definitely possible. While this list of herbs and vegetables does remarkably well with little water in high heat, they cannot live *without* water and still need regular moisture.

- Amaranth
- Asparagus
- Broccoli
- Cabbage
- Chards
- Chinese cabbage
- Dandelion
- German chamomile
- Lavender
- Leeks
- Malabar spinach
- Onions
- Oregano
- Peppers
- Rhubarb
- Rosemary
- Sage
- Squash
- Thyme
- Tomatoes
- Winter savory

KITCHEN GARDEN TIPS

- It is assumed that all the foods used in your kitchen garden will be consumed by your family, so growing organically is absolutely critical to reduce chemical exposure.
- Potager gardens perform best when receiving full sun, or six to eight hours of sun per day. However, it is possible to grow vegetables in shade (see box on page 68).
- Vegetables and herbs need to be rotated seasonally, and the soil needs to be replenished by adding plenty of compost and new material annually.
- Mulch your gardens to keep weeds back and hold in moisture.
- Vegetables, fruits, and herbs need more water. For lower maintenance watering, install a drip system in the garden.
- Do research with all plants you put in your kitchen garden to make sure they are safe. For example, do not plant poisonous plants, which might harm a person upon consumption.

Succession planting helps you harvest more food. If a plant has stopped producing or has been harvested, try planting a new row of seeds or throw in a new plant to stretch out the seasonal food production.

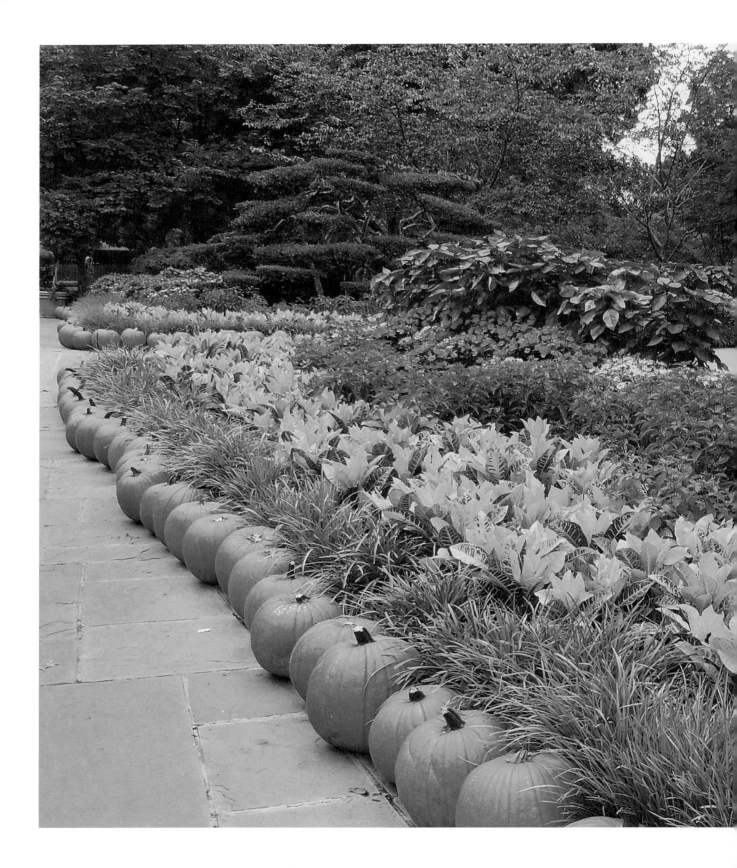

PART II

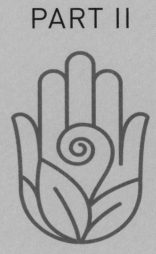

INCORPORATING EXERCISE IN THE GARDEN

To be effective, exercise in the garden does not have to be extreme or strenuous. Walking outdoors in the fresh air is a light exercise that you can enjoy at your own pace in your own yard or garden. Intentional walks in parks or public gardens like the Dallas Arboretum and Botanical Gardens can be incredibly stress relieving and refreshing to the soul. A daily walk can be a beautiful and mindful way to exercise.

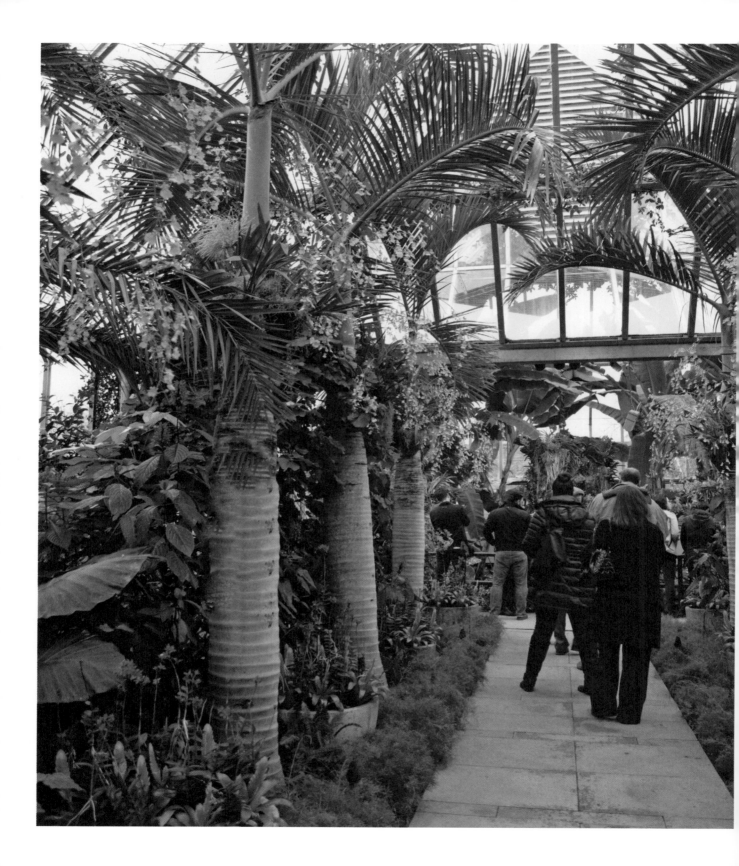

6

WALKING IN THE GREEN

MODERATE EXERCISE IS necessary for good health and is particularly effective in reducing stress symptoms and alleviating depression and anxiety. Gardening can certainly be considered "moderate exercise" if thoughtfully performed, and getting outside a little every day in the garden can be an important part of the wellness lifestyle plan. More importantly, connecting a daily moderate exercise to our regimen can make us happier.

In some areas of the world, people can garden every day of the year, but in other zones, gardening is restricted during the winter season. With this in mind, I recommend coming up with a combination exercise plan of organic gardening activities and walking regularly to get yourself out of your home and away from the computer and television. Consult with your medical professional and build a plan together. My plan, which was suggested by my osteoarthritis surgeon, my physical therapist, and my nutritionist, was simple to begin with: walk one hour every day, whether inside or outside.

Chris Powell, trainer and exercise science expert, says in his book *Choose to Lose*, "People who make exercise a priority have lower rates of cancer, heart disease, and high blood pressure.

OPPOSITE: Rainy weather got you down? Consider walking at greenhouses or nurseries where you can continue to get a lot of exposure to plants and oxygenated air. Local shopping malls and department stores also offer large interior spaces to walk. The point is to keep moving. *Photo taken at Chicago Botanic Garden.*

More oxygen is available to every organ of their body, and their muscles are stronger. Regular exercisers have lower rates of depression and other mental disorders. They have more energy and feel better than non-exercisers." Going from a person who only gardened seasonally, to a person who walks daily and gardens seasonally, I can tell you that I have seen a tremendous reduction in pain and increase in overall wellness.

HEART RATE AND EXERCISE

Tracking your heart rate can help you better understand your physical health. Typically, the resting heart rate of an average adult ranges from 60 to 100 beats per minute. Use a digital tracker or learn how to take your heart rate (see below) and start documenting your regular heart beat at rest: it will help you determine your progress.

When the heart rate is at rest and is lower, the heart is functioning more efficiently. Having a lower heart rate can also help determine cardiovascular fitness. Many professional athletes can have a resting heart rate of 40 beats per minute, which is indeed exceptionally low but reflects their intense cardiovascular-focused exercise program.

How to Take Your Resting Heart Rate

A *resting heart rate* is the measurement of the number of times your heart beats per minute while you are resting. Perhaps the most convenient time to check your resting heart rate is before you get out of bed in the morning.

Find your pulse on the inside of your wrists on the thumb side, inside your elbow, on the side of your neck below your ear, or at the top of your foot. Put your finger on the pulse point and count how many beats there are in one minute.

The result will be your resting heart rate. Tracking your resting rate can help you better understand your cardiovascular health and assist with exercise target heart rates.

HOW TO TAKE AND TRACK YOUR EXERCISING HEART RATE

Training heart rates are heart rates measured during exercise. Occasionally stop during your gardening or walking exercise and take your pulse. A shortcut method to take your pulse during exercise is to count your pulse for only 10 seconds and multiply by 6 to find an approximate beat per minute result.

Your **maximum training heart rate** is about 220 minus your age. If an individual is 40 years old, for example, he would subtract 40 from 220 to get the result of 180 beats per minute: that is his average maximum heart rate (220 − 40 = 180).

Your **target heart rate** ranges from 50 to 85 percent of your maximum heart rate. Continuing with the example of the 40-year-old, his target heart rate zone would be 90 to 153 beats per minute.

According to the American Heart Association's website, "If your heart rate is too high, you're straining. So, slow down. If it's too low, and the intensity feels 'light' or 'moderate/brisk,' you may want to push yourself to exercise a little harder. During the first few weeks of working out, aim for the lower ranger of your target zone [50 percent] and gradually build up to the higher range [85 percent]. After six months or more, you may be able to exercise comfortably at up to 85 percent of your maximum heart rate."

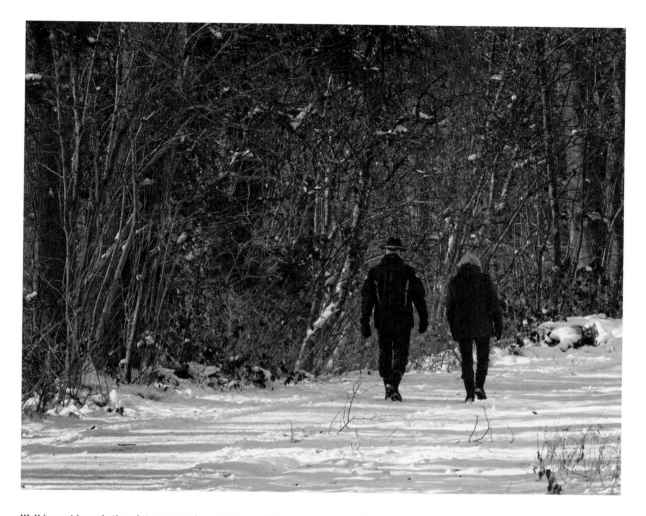

Walking outdoors in the winter season is as vital as walking in the summer. If you have a health condition that requires steadier footing, walking on winter trails might not be an option. However, it is important to walk daily whenever possible to keep your joints, muscles, and system fluid. Walking, even at a very slow pace, is better than not walking at all. Be sure to check with your health care providers before starting a regular walking program.

When I first began my walking program, my average resting heart rate ranged from 89 to a surprisingly dismal 95. After one year of gardening whenever I was able and walking daily, my resting heart rate improved to about 69 to 75 beats per minute. That's good progress made with moderate exercise.

An advantage of walking regularly is that it is convenient and free. You do not have to buy into an expensive health club to exercise for 20 or 30 minutes every day. Instead, you can step right outside your front door and achieve excellent results. Exercising out in nature gives you energy and lifts your spirits as well.

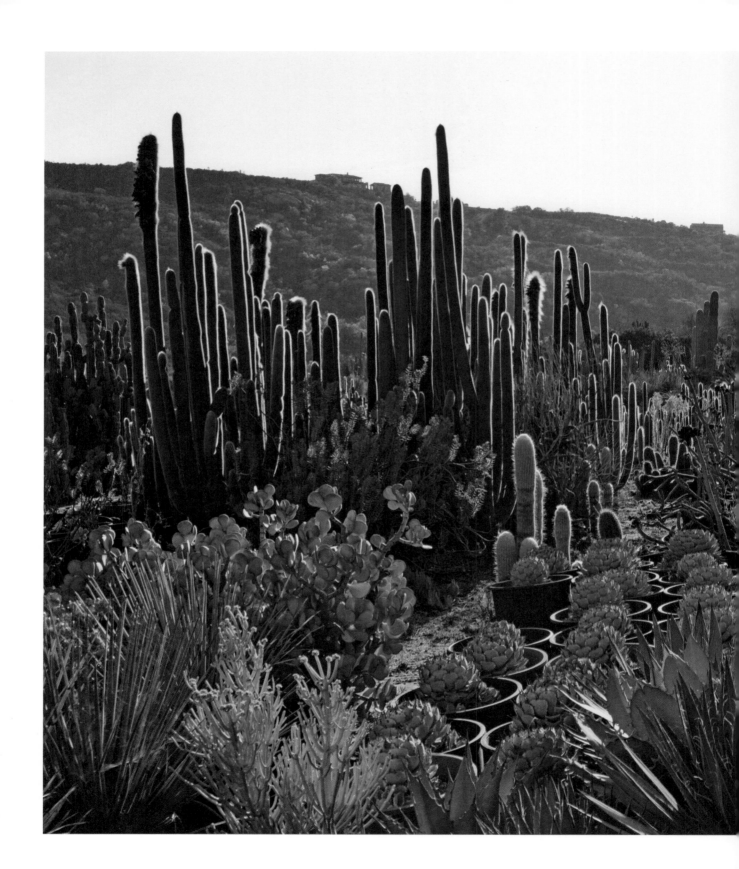

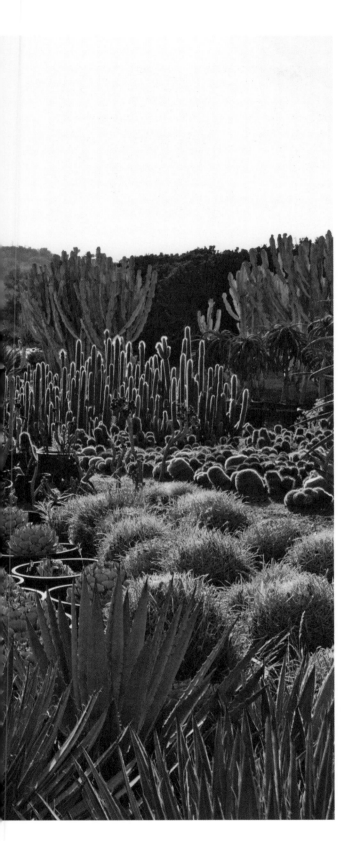

When I first began walking daily, my degenerative osteoarthritis pain was so great that I could barely walk 1,000 steps in an hour. I joined a local health club for a while and walked inside during the extreme heat of summer, and I cried like a baby every day and with every step. Each step, however, helped me come closer to less inflammation and less pain. Diet helped immensely as well, and the combination of the anti-inflammatory diet with daily exercise was tremendously beneficial.

As time progressed, my daily gardening and walking adventures helped strengthen me. Sometimes when I walked, I wrote books or blog posts in my head, so that while my body was occupied, my mind was as well. At other times, I would drift in thought and mind in an almost meditative state. Now, several years from when I first began, I typically walk about 5,000 to 6,000 steps per hour.

When you begin your walking program, be sure to start slow and get your doctor's recommendation on a walking and exercise plan that works for you. Track your heart rate and make sure you're not straining or pushing too hard. Slow down, think, breathe, and experience gardens, fresh air, and sunshine as often as you possibly can. It's a daily journey that will become uplifting to the mind and body.

Looking for a creative and fun place to walk? A great way to get in touch with plants and be outside in the fresh air is to try walking at garden nurseries and garden centers. This image shows the astoundingly beautiful Desert Theater Nursery in Escondido, California; its cactus and succulent plants are world famous. Exploring a nursery is a great way to get your daily steps in and also see fabulous plants in large groupings. Seeing all those plants is truly a delightful way to help you plan your gardens while maintaining your health.

FINDING HAPPINESS

One of the immensely wonderful benefits of both walking and gardening outside is a physical and emotional response described as "flow" by a psychology professor, Mihaly Csikszentmihalyi, PhD (pronounced *Me-high Cheek-sent-me-high*. He wrote *Flow: The Psychology of Optimal Experience*. In that book, he reflects on his passion to learn more about the process of human enjoyment and documents what he describes as a condition called "flow." Flow is the pleasurable sensation of losing oneself in an activity—work, a game, gardening, or a physical or mental challenge—and becoming immersed, with everything perfectly meshing in a harmonious state where goals are set and satisfyingly met. Flow is an experience between concentrated focus on a goal and a feeling of mechanical effortlessness. Time contracts or stretches, and the individual merges with the action, totally absorbed.

What he learned is that work can be as emotionally satisfying as play. This is why some people feel frustrated when they retire from their job: they have lost a consistent schedule in their days that enable them to concentrate and work toward a goal. Feeling useful, feeling active, and feeling emotionally content are all tied together in the principles of Professor Csikszentmihalyi's "flow" concept. He writes in his book *The Evolving Self*, "Contrary to expectation, 'flow' usually happens not during relaxing moments of leisure and entertainment, but rather when we are actively involved in a difficult enterprise, in a task that stretches our mental and physical abilities."

He continues, "It turns out that when challenges are high and personal skills are used

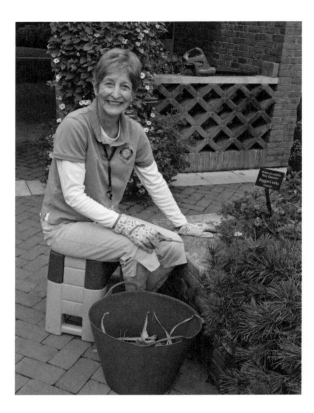

Happiness is that amazing feeling of immersing yourself in an activity like gardening, which combines a satisfying activity with a sense of accomplishment. Activities like this can help reduce depression and increase a positive mental state. Here we see a volunteer at the Chicago Botanic Garden tending the elevated garden beds in the Beuhler Enabling Garden. *Photo taken at Chicago Botanic Garden.*

to the utmost, we experience this rare state of consciousness. The first symptom of flow is a narrowing of attention on a clearly defined goal. We feel involved, concentrated, absorbed. We know what must be done, and we get immediate feedback as to how well we are doing. The tennis player knows after each shot whether the ball actually went where she wanted it to go; the pianist knows after each stroke of the keyboard whether the notes sound like they should. Even a usually boring job, once the challenges are brought into balance with the person's skills and the goals are clarified, can begin to be exciting and involving. . . . Often we feel a sense of transcendence, as if the boundaries of the self had been expanded. The sailor feels at one with the wind, the boat, and the sea; the singer feels a mysterious sense of universal harmony. In those moments the awareness of time disappears, and hours seem to flash by without our noticing. This state of consciousness . . . comes as close as anything can to what we call happiness."

What is critical to outdoor walking and green exercises is Csikszentmihalyi's definition of a "sense of transcendence" that happens when performing these activities. This explains what happens to me while I am walking and is often the experience I have while gardening. The feeling can easily happen to anyone who spends time outside walking and gardening regularly. In fact, many people who are in the garden doing repetitive work discover this since of wellness. This is why some say that "weeding is therapy." Repetitive work develops a sense of flow as much as a more specifically creative activity. Flow requires effort. Flow is not "wasting time," but is instead being present and active in the moment, and definitively represents the feeling of happiness and contentment.

NOT CONVINCED YET?

Committing to walking every day is, without a doubt, a challenge from a time perspective. Unlike going to a club or paying for a class, it does not have the "guilt" motivation of wasted money if you do not show up. You have to keep the end in mind: the benefits your new wellness lifestyle will bring you.

According to the Arthritis Foundation (AF), there are several clear benefits of walking for all people, but especially for people suffering from arthritis. The AF reports that walking can also improve memory and slow mental decline. "A study of 6,000 women, ages 65 and older, performed by researchers at the University of California, San Francisco, found that age-related memory decline was lower in those who walked more. The women walking 2.5 miles per day had a 17 percent decline in memory, as opposed to a 25 percent decline in women who walked less than a half-mile per week." Walking also improves circulation, makes bones stronger, increases lifespan, improves mood, can lead to weight loss, strengthens muscles, improves sleep, supports joint fluid to joints, increases oxygen levels, reduces Alzheimer's risk, and most significantly improves circulation and lowers blood pressure.

When I was diagnosed with severe degenerative spinal osteoarthritis, I found it difficult to stand upright. Yet, walking—at my own pace—soon helped me regain my posture and lose much of the chronic pain. Walk slowly for the first 8 to 10 minutes to let your system warm up. Then speed up to a stronger walk. Cool down at the end of your walk by again walking more slowly for an additional 8 to 10 minutes. My physical therapists recommend that I stretch gently after the walk or after the 10-minute warm-up to improve my joint flexibility, but not before. Please consult with your medical professionals for their best advice.

When you walk, concentrate on keeping your back straight and head up. Swing your arms comfortably. While a small amount of "arm pumping" is okay, if you have a physical condition or injury, the pumping action can inflame your injury. Therefore, take it slow to start. Walk with your stomach muscles tightened a bit and smoothly roll your feet as you move.

Even on the days I felt challenged to complete my walk, I persisted and walked an hour. Some days that might mean I would barely hover at 1,000 steps per hour and other days, when my pain began to ease, I achieved 6,000 steps or more per hour. What helped me get through the walks was giving myself something to observe while I was on the move. My best recommendation is good old Mother Nature—walk through gardens, nature preserves, and arboretums, or even down a tree-lined street. When I cannot walk outside due to inclement weather, I walk the local grocery store or shopping mall.

Get started walking right away. Begin by tracking your heart rate. This will allow you to see positive progress. Combined with gardening and diet, you can lower blood pressure, improve your health, reduce your pain, and feel so much better.

As important as walking is to your health, many struggle to walk for longer lengths of time without a break. Public gardens like Chanticleer in Wayne, Pennsylvania, offer regular seating for visitors. Here you see a rambling plant bed at the Ruin Garden, yet it has firm and secure footing and a comfortable seat for anyone who needs a rest. Plan seating into your own gardens to help you on your walks and regular exercise adventures.

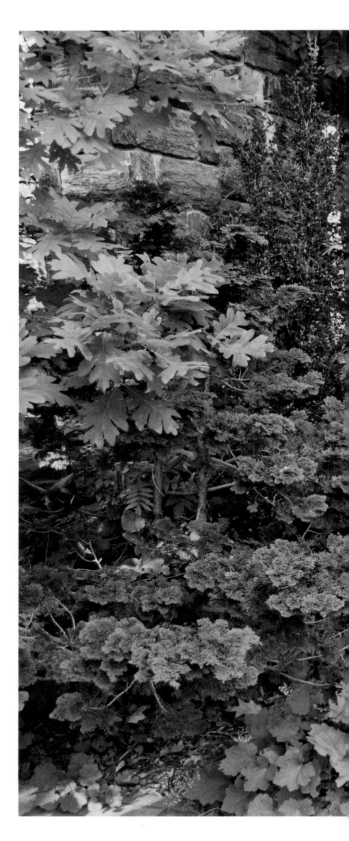

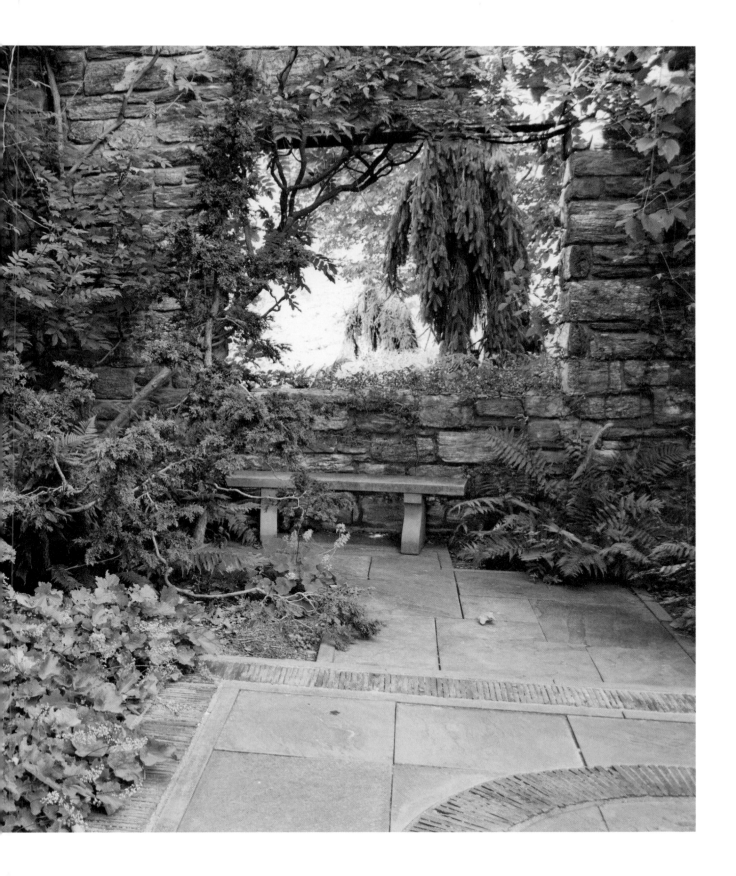

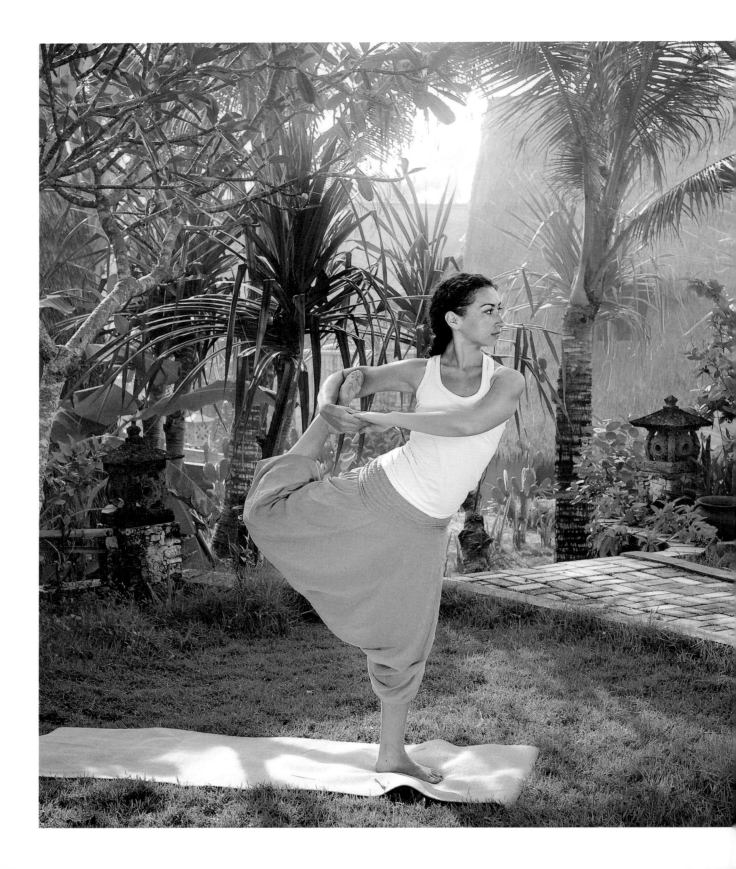

7

YOGA IN THE GARDEN

PHYSICAL EXERCISE IN the garden provides exposure to the outdoors and enhances mental flow experiences. This can help you reach a more physical and emotional state of wellness. Exercise can include repetitive activities like weeding, digging, planting, mowing, walking, and building. However, it should be noted that exceptionally strenuous work in the garden is not necessary to feel good: in fact, it can lead to injuries. Care must be taken, particularly if you have an injury or limiting physical condition.

THE STRESS EFFECT

OPPOSITE: Being outdoors while you are doing any exercise enhances your physical and mental health. Yoga practice, in particular, can be improved with an outdoor connection because of the dedicated breathing needed to perform the exercise. Breathing fresh air deeply is energizing.
Mazan Xeniya/Shutterstock.

There are many reasons exercise is important for good health, and combatting stress is one of those reasons. Stress has become a serious modern societal issue. Stressors in our high-paced lives may include family and relationships, money issues, pressures at work, and complicated political-economic-governmental issues that upset our emotions and natural routines.

Exercise, and yoga specifically, is a great outlet for the energies related to anger and hostility and can help reduce stress-related illnesses such as gastrointestinal problems, heart disease, high blood

RIGHT: Yoga is a particularly effective exercise to remove stress. General benefits of yoga include increased muscle strength and tone, increased flexibility, improved stress reduction, enhanced cardio and circulatory health, enriched breathing, and higher energy levels. Practicing yoga outdoors at every opportunity helps improve mood as well. *Dreamer Company/Shutterstock.*

BELOW: Practicing yoga with friends in your garden can be a social experience that brings your neighbors together to connect with wellness. Jenny Peterson, Terri Curtis, and Jacque Gregory (left to right) perform yoga on Jenny's yoga deck in Austin, Texas, sharing time and health together.

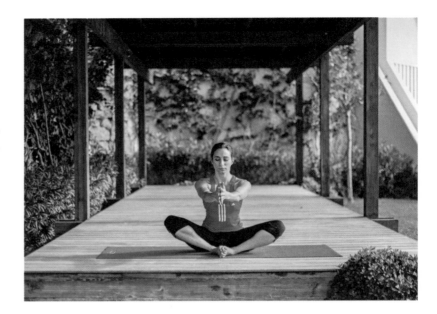

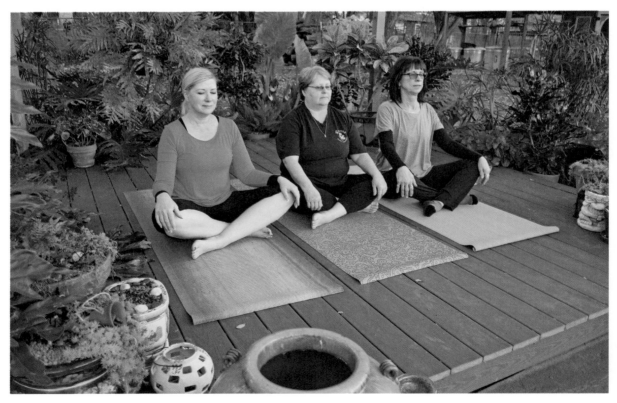

pressure, obesity, asthma, diabetes, circulation issues, fibromyalgia, chronic pain, depression, and insomnia. Used properly, all exercise provides a socially acceptable means of physically releasing negative energy.

Most specifically, endorphins have been shown to increase during physical activity of 20 minutes or more. Therefore, it is important to walk, garden, or do another activity such as yoga, for more than 20 minutes at a time several times per week. Chemically comparable to opiate compounds, endorphins are similar to morphine-like substances and have been shown to provide a pain-relieving effect and promote a sense of euphoria.

THE BENEFITS OF YOGA

Yoga is a particularly effective way to help your body and mind feel well and encourage stress reduction. Many people assume yoga is only about stretching and movement, but it is far more than that as its roots are set deeply in the Hindu religion and are centered on cultivating mental mindfulness. To be clear, yoga is not a religion, but is instead a philosophical and physical practice. Definitively the word *yoga* is often defined as "union" and is known as an ascetic discipline that combines meditation, breath control, and physical body postures to help attain stamina, physical strength, and overall better health.

Daphne Miller, MD, author of *Farmacology*, writes, "Ancient contemplative techniques such as meditation and yoga have also been shown to increase self-esteem and reverse the chronic negative effects of stress. . . . These pursuits cultivate compassion and kindness, two positive emotions that seem to play a key role in shrinking the amygdala (the anxiety center) and increasing the size of the hippocampus [in the brain]. Not surprisingly, studies show that experienced practitioners of mindfulness show more [brain] plasticity than those who occasionally say a couple 'ohms.'"

Nearly 2,000 years ago, an Indian scholar, Patanjali, assembled the practice of yoga into the *Yoga Sutra*, which is a collection of statements that serves as the basis for much of the yoga as it is practiced in modern day. There are many types of yoga practiced today, and participants often describe the experience of learning yoga as very mentally and physically self-transformational.

The "ohm" that Daphne Miller, MD, mentions in the paragraph above refers to the traditional mantra, or vibration, that is often chanted at the beginning and the end of yoga sessions. This vibration is meant to encourage better breathing, center awareness, and help a person connect more intimately with the yoga experience. It is highly recommended that you attend yoga classes in order to effectively learn the proper poses or postures. However, you can learn yoga on your own.

Inspired by the principle of yoga, I took several classes, then began seeking my own path by reading books, practicing with cell phone apps, and consulting the experts whenever possible. My favorite time to perform yoga is on my lunch hour. This is a time when I need a bit of an energy break from the stresses of working on the computer, and since I work out of my home, I am able to take a yoga break in my garden.

GARDEN YOGA

Yoga is often practiced indoors, of course. But performing yoga outdoors, in nature or in the garden, can be immensely stimulating and joyful.

Jenny Peterson, author of *The Cancer Survivor's Garden Companion* has a beautiful yoga platform in her back garden. As a cancer survivor, she credits the yoga as an essential daily health gift that has helped her stay well and cancer free. Every morning Jenny gets up and spends the first part of her morning performing yoga in her garden. "After my cancer treatment," she says,

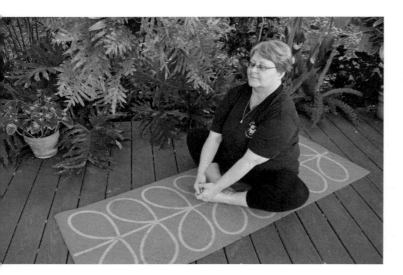

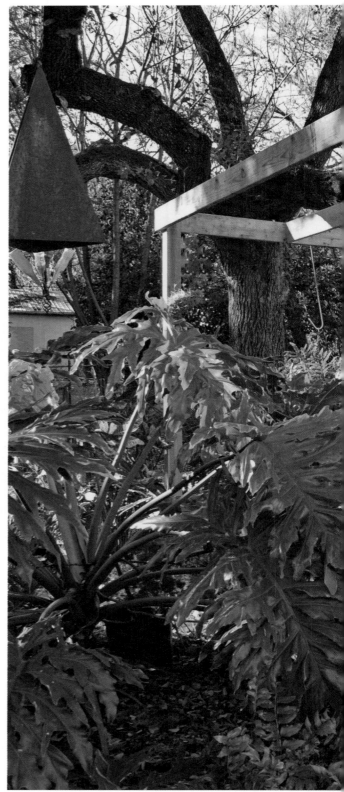

ABOVE: Terri Curtis relaxes into a pose on Jenny Peterson's unique garden yoga platform in Austin, Texas, surrounded by nature and plants.

RIGHT: Jenny Peterson's astoundingly cool yoga platform raises the yoga practice above the soil level in an open area in the backyard. You can see her chicken house and goat pen in the background, so she has surrounded the platform with gorgeous plants that make her feel relaxed and happy. Jenny, author of *The Cancer Survivor's Garden Companion* and a cancer survivor herself, brings her coffee out in the morning and does daily yoga as an emotional and physical health relief.

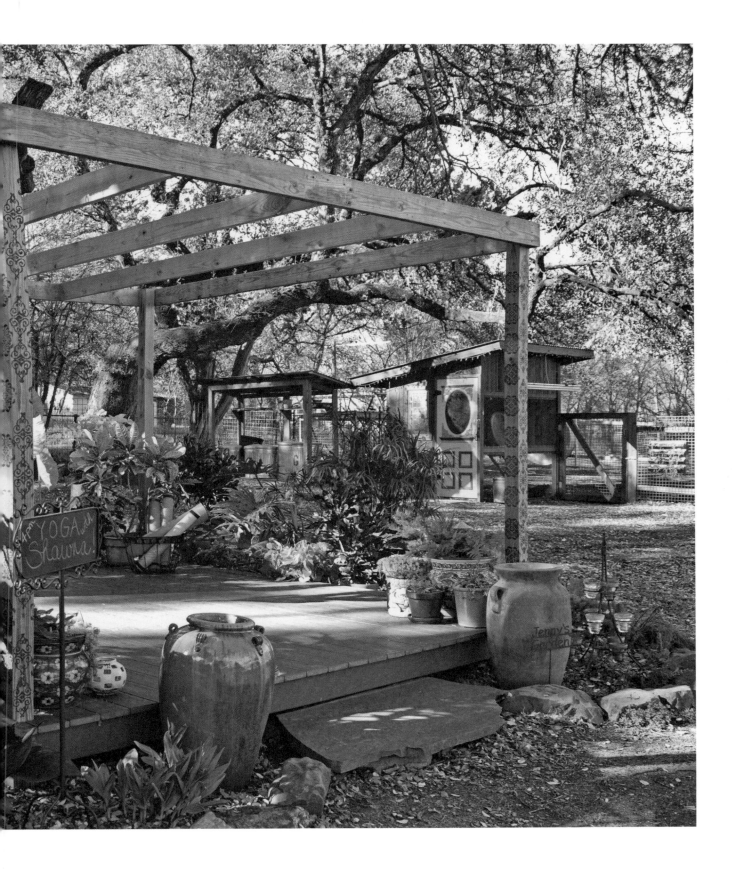

"I had lymphedema, nerve damage in my feet, and lots of scar tissue that created range of motion issues for me, and even depression. I'd always loved yoga and knew how healing it was, so my husband built me a yoga deck in our backyard to help me get back on track. We've since created a lush tropical garden around it—I hear birds chirping, feel the breeze blowing, inhale the scents—it's like the garden is surrounding me and saying, 'It's going to be okay, Jenny.'"

Creating your garden yoga space takes some forethought to create a quiet, healing haven.

- Create a comfortable space. Gardens are filled with insects, moisture, and work waiting to be completed. Your yoga area needs to have less distractions—like wet ground or biting bugs—and more peace. Whether you select a patio or grassy area, it needs to be flat so that you can do your poses comfortably, in private, and in an area with minimal distraction.
- Think therapy. Placing your yoga space near a garden area that inspires you, smells delicious because of herbs or plants, or simply makes you happy is an excellent idea. If you like where you are in the garden, it will bring more therapeutic benefits to you as you will want to come back often to experience that same beauty and peace.
- Bring your mat. Practicing yoga on a mat enables you to have a barrier of protection from soil, rocks, and unforgiving concrete. Cushioned yoga mats make doing poses more comfortable. Do not leave the mat outside as it can be damaged by weather. Instead, bring the mat outdoors as you would if you are having a formal class; roll it up and store it until next time.

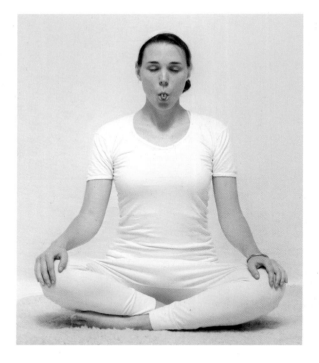

Yogic breathing may feel a little uncomfortable at first, but it truly works as an effective calming technique. Practice sitali pranayama by sitting up and crossing your legs, back straight, and arms relaxed. Shape your tongue like a straw, bringing the sides of your tongue up, then stick your tongue slightly out of your mouth. Slowly inhale a deep breath. At the very end of your deep inhale, put your tongue back to its normal position, close your mouth, and exhale slowly. Practice for 20 breaths this technique of inhaling and slowly exhaling. *Gurudayal Khalsa Photography.*

One of the benefits of practicing yoga in the garden is that fresh air surrounds you, plus being in an open space can enrich your yogic breathing. Proper breathing technique is an important component of yoga and is sometimes a challenge for beginning yoga participants. When we position ourselves into a particular pose, the tendency is to hold the breath. Unfortunately, this builds stress in the body and causes tension.

Yogic breathing is known as *pranayama*: it emphasizes having a calm body with regular breathing as you move through the flowing sequence of postures. There are many different types of breathing techniques that are dependent on the specific posture being held, so it can be helpful to have a teacher or guide work with you while you are learning.

When tense or stressed, humans breathe more shallowly. Pranayama helps you to disrupt your emotional stress and shallow breathing pattern by enabling a change in the way you inhale and exhale. Your breathing transforms into long breaths that are even and full.

BREATHING PRACTICE

Try a standard deep breathing technique: start by lying down on the floor with knees bent and eyes closed. Put your hand on your tummy, near your belly button, and take several deep, calming breaths. Feel how your breath makes your abdomen expand and contract. This deep breathing moves your diaphragm and enables your lungs to capture more oxygen. Practice this technique for 15 breaths.

Next, practice *sitali pranayama*, which is known as "the cooling breath." It has the ability to improve focus and reduce anxiety. Sit up and cross your legs, with back straight and arms relaxed. Shape your tongue like a straw, bringing the sides of your tongue up, then stick your tongue slightly out of your mouth. Slowly inhale a deep breath; you may or may not hear your breath.

If you cannot curl your tongue, you can try a slightly different technique known as *sitkari pranayama*: simply press your lower and upper teeth together and separate your lips so that you can take in breath through the gaps in your teeth. Inhale slowly through the gaps in your teeth, making a slight hissing sound as you take a deep breath.

At the very end of your inhale for either the sitali pranayama or the sitkari pranayama, put your tongue back to its normal position, close your mouth, and exhale slowly. Practice for 20 breaths your chosen method of inhaling and slowly exhaling.

Another technique in breathing is a long exhale. In this practice, you want your exhale to be twice as long as your inhale. This technique can be performed in the sitting or standing position and is particularly effective for sleeping issues if done in bed, lying down, before sleep. Begin by practicing your standard deep breathing technique for a few breaths. When you feel relaxed, slowly increase the exhalation by a few seconds every breath until you double the length of the exhale as compared to the length of your inhale. If you are gasping or short of breath, you are being too aggressive about the exhale without a strong enough inhale. Make it long, calm, and slow.

These techniques might feel unusual at first, but with practice it is quite effective. In fact, these techniques are exceptionally calming and can work very well to help stressed individuals sleep better, whether they are used in yoga or simply as a quiet exercise. Although these breathing techniques are inherently used in yoga, they are also wonderful to experience as you are standing, sitting, or laying outdoors in the garden. In my experience, it helps to connect you to the garden and nature in a uniquely calming way.

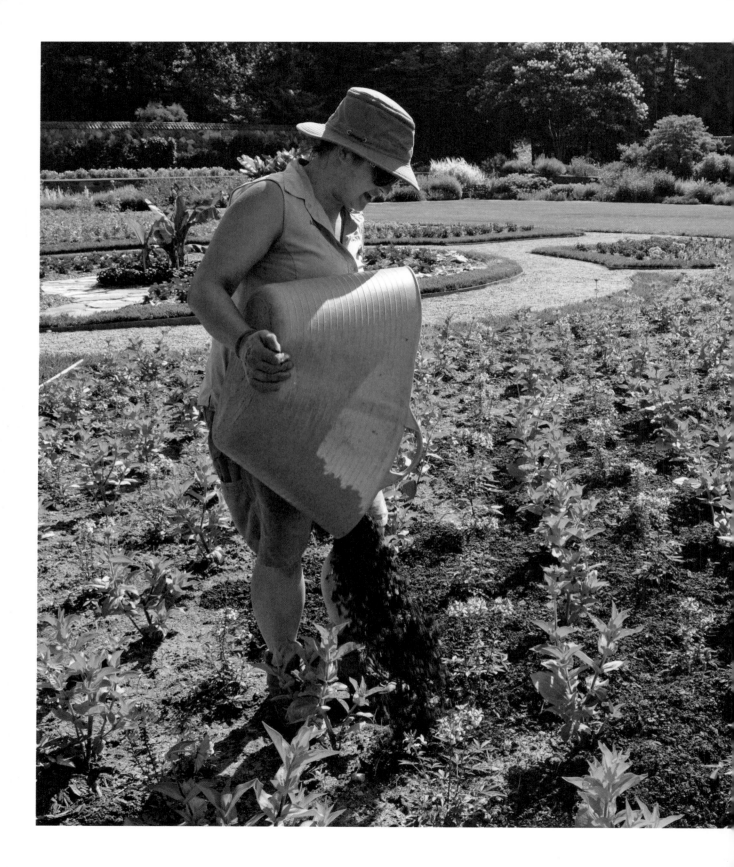

8

EXERCISE IN THE GARDEN

EXERCISE IS IMPORTANT for all humans, but is particularly critical for people who suffer inflammatory conditions. According to the United States National Library of Medicine–National Institutes of Health, many studies have demonstrated that cardiovascular exercise can reduce markers of systemic inflammation in all people, but particularly for the elderly. Knowing that chronic pain is often connected with inflammation, it makes sense to continue with a cardiovascular exercise program.

Warming up is important as well, especially when working in the garden. According to the US National Library of Medicine–National Institutes of Health 1998 study, more than 2.1 million people were injured doing gardening or yard work in the 30 days of the study. The survey results report, "During walking and gardening, men and women were equally likely to be injured, but younger people (18–44 yr) were more likely to be injured than older people (45 + yr). . . . large numbers of people were injured because participation rates were high. Most injuries were minor, but injuries may reduce participation in these otherwise beneficial activities."

OPPOSITE: Exercising properly as a part of doing daily or weekly garden maintenance can truly enhance your health, particularly for those who suffer inflammatory conditions. Make sure that you do not overextend your muscles, inflame joints, or injure yourself as a part of that exercise. Here a professional gardener at Biltmore Estate in Asheville, North Carolina, mulches, lifting and pouring from a small, flexible container in order to lighten her load and reduce strain on her back.

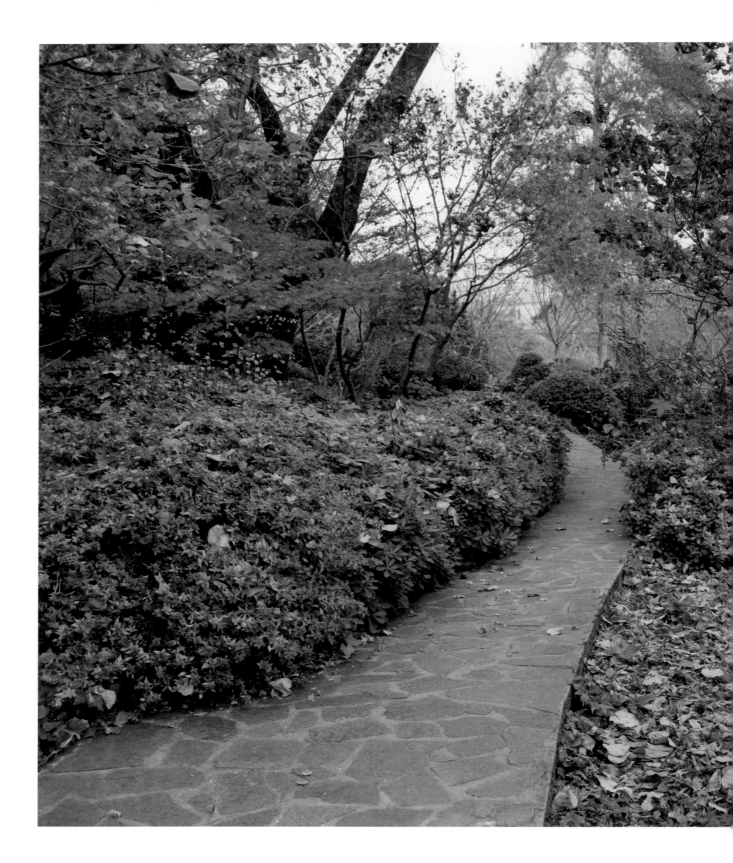

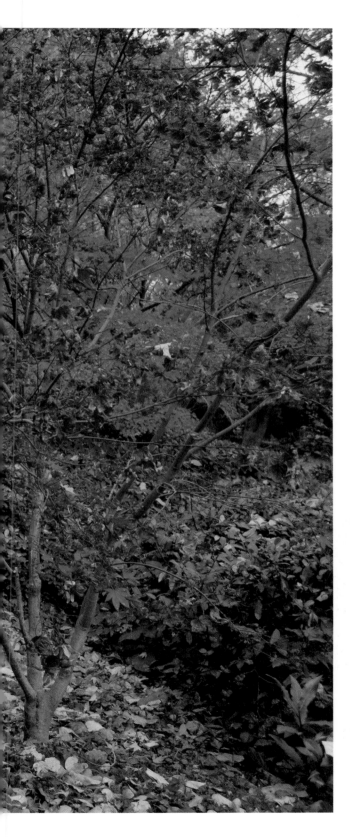

We might hypothesize that the reason people under the age of 45 are being injured more often is because they are attempting to do heavier work and lifting. However, improper use of equipment along with repetitive motions can also cause many injuries, some of which could have been prevented with simple warm-up exercises.

THE WARM-UP

One of the reasons warming up is so important is that it helps you identify if something is wrong. Do you feel pain in an unusual spot? Do you find it difficult to do certain movements? Do you feel out of breath and you just started warming up? Do you feel dizzy? These are all signs that it might be wise to avoid heavy gardening and yard mowing that day—stop what you are doing—and go get checked out by a health professional.

Warming up properly gradually increases your cardiovascular system's activities so that you are raising temperatures in your body slowly, making your joints and muscles more workable and increasing blood flow to your muscles at an even pace. The simplest warm-up includes walking, but based on your health care professional's recommendation, a warm-up might also include a series of gentle rotations of head, forearms, arms, shoulders, torso, hips, knees, and feet. A simple warm-up could be to briskly walk for

This beautiful garden path can be found at Orto Botanico in Rome, Italy. Garden paths, forested areas, or even your neighborhood sidewalk represents places you use for a quick warm-up before heavier exercise. Medical professionals agree that warming up can help reduce injury. So, find your path—or sidewalk—and spend 10 minutes walking before your garden chores.

about 10 minutes before performing physical gardening chores.

If you feel walking does not get your heart pumping as much as you would like, incorporate more dynamic or active exercises into your warm-up such as jumping jacks, marching, knee bending, front leg swings, and side bends. Along with warming up, various exercises can activate specific muscles you will use during your workout and reduce damage. Should you have an injury, joint disorder, or physical limitation, it is particularly important to ask your doctor before undertaking a more active warm-up and exercise routine. Whether slow or more active, warming up is important to your physical health, particularly if you suffer from an injury or disability that makes gardening more challenging.

STRETCHING BENEFITS
JOINT RANGE OF MOTION

Stretching can be important but not for the reasons you may have suspected. New evidence shows that static stretching is not an effective warm-up, nor does it prevent injury. Len Kravitz, PhD, of The University of New Mexico, reports in his research article, "Stretching: A Research Retrospective," that stretching does not prevent injury or delayed onset muscle soreness in exercise. "Perhaps one of the most exhaustive and comprehensive research reviews on the impact of stretching and sport injury risk . . . [said] that pre-exercise stretching does not prevent injury among competitive or recreational athletes . . . studies [demonstrate that] incorporating a pre-exercise combination of resistance exercise, body conditioning, and warm-up show promise for better injury prevention."

With this in mind, active stretching should not happen before your body is warmed up, and indeed, should probably happen at the end of the gardening or exercise activity. Stretching does not lessen injury or post-exercise pain.

If stretching does not prevent injury or help with muscle soreness, what's the point of it? At the top of my list is something simple—it feels good. There are also medically helpful reasons to

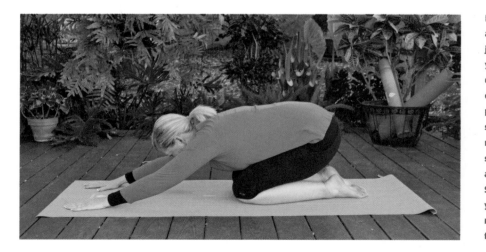

Increasing range of motion is a good thing to do if you have joint concerns. Stretching like yoga expert Jenny Peterson is doing here can enhance range of motion; however, it's been proven through numerous studies that stretching does not prevent injury. Stretches should be done after you are already warmed up. Stretching is a great tool if you have a joint condition but might not be the first choice for pre-aerobic exercise.

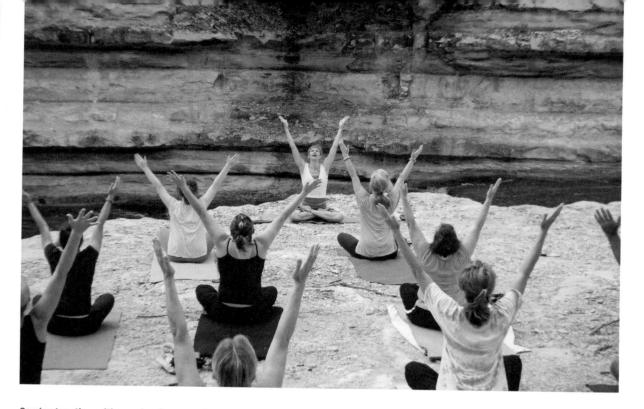

Coming together with your local community in a guided exercise class with an experienced instructor can give you guidance for your specific physical needs. Research local classes that might be held outdoors or at botanical gardens to connect with new friends focused on wellness. *Public Domain Pixabay.com.*

stretch; for example, many of the people suffering arthropathic diseases such as rheumatoid arthritis and osteoarthritis have decreased joint mobility and often feel stiff and unable to move without suffering inflammatory pain. Including stretching exercises in an exercise routine if you have such problems can help increase mobility and flexibility, which helps to reduce chronic pain. Stretching regularly after your body is warmed up helps to maintain long-term flexibility benefits as well.

EXPERTS TO GUIDE YOU

While it would be lovely if we could all have an exercise expert with us in the garden to advise

what's best for our individual conditions, this is rarely practical. If you are suffering physical discomfort with joints or muscles, consider consulting a specialist such as a physiatrist, orthopedist, or rheumatologist to help you get a better handle on your physical health. They will recommend a course of action that includes a series of exercises best suited to your needs. Perhaps you have no specific limiting physical condition. In that case, your expert consultant might be an exercise instructor at a local gym or fitness center.

Should you have a limiting physical condition, then follow the exercise advice of your doctor.

Tips to Get Motivated to Exercise

Exercising such as walking, stretching, or yoga can be a challenge to fit into our day; we have busy lives and it can be difficult to make the time to do the physical exercise that is so very important to the wellness lifestyle. Below are a few tips that might help you stay on track with your daily exercise goals.

- **Find your happy place.** Whenever possible, exercise in the garden, at a park, or somewhere you enjoy the view and outdoor experience. Do research and find all the beautiful places near your home and make sure you go to explore them by walking whenever possible.
- **Schedule it.** Write down the time and hour of your exercise in your calendar and treat it like a business or medical appointment; arrive on time and be ready to do the work necessary. Do not miss your appointment.
- **Involve friends and family.** Exercise with friends or family if you struggle to stay committed by yourself. Encouragement in a team atmosphere can make all the difference.
- **Document everything.** Keep a log of your activity and progress. This is particularly important because it helps you see how far you have come from the time you started your plan.
- **Sign on the dotted line.** Often we promise ourselves we are going to dedicate more time to our health and quickly fall off of the program. However, it has been shown through studies that people who made a verbal or written commitment in front of friends and family were more likely to follow through with their exercise program. It is embarrassing to fall off of the plan when others are sticking with it. Additionally, some make a financial commitment such as, "For every day of walking missed, I commit to pay $5 to my friend," or "For every day of walking missed, I must do the dishes after the family dinner." Create and sign a contract with your friends or family pledging that you will commit to walking daily for six months.
- **Plan for rewards.** A self-motivation trick that has worked for me is to reward yourself when you reach goals. For example, if you meet your goal of walking every day for 30 days, perhaps you can give yourself permission to have a little "bonus" fun at the end of the time period. Reward yourself by joining a class, buying a new gardening or cooking book, visiting the library, having a spa day, seeing a movie in the theater, buying a bouquet of flowers, going to a museum for an afternoon, or packing a picnic lunch and enjoying your favorite garden for a few hours.

Reach out to an experienced yoga instructor or physical therapist so they can teach you stretches and exercises that are most likely to help you improve your condition and strengthen your joints and body.

They might also recommend that you first join a class in tai chi or yoga. These classes are often held outside in a garden or park and offer the benefits of group participation and a guided process with a certified instructor.

FLARE-UPS AND SORENESS

Poor posture and walking issues are often attributed to chronic inflammatory conditions such as arthritis, yet many of these issues are formed initially due to inactivity. Remaining active and keeping your joints and muscles fluid is the key to prevention. According to *Arthritis: What Exercises Work*, by Dava Sobel and Arthur C. Klein, "As we discovered while doing research . . . exercise helped 95 percent of those Arthritis Survey participants

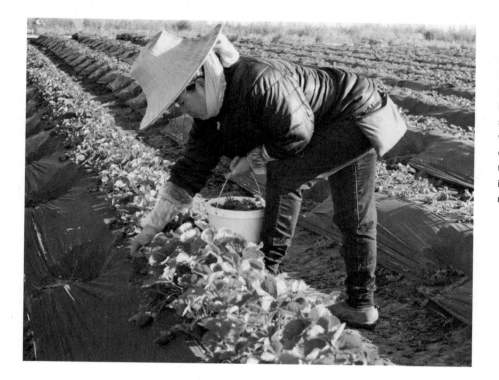

When bending or doing other exercises in the garden, particularly if you have a concern with back pain, be sure to lift up one leg to give you additional support in the bend. Consult with a physical therapist or medical professional to better understand your individual concerns and needs related to exercise.

who tried it. No other approach to arthritis—no drug, no surgical procedure—matches exercise for high rates of improvement. Nor can any other treatment modality boast exercise's low risk of serious complications or unpleasant side effects."

Anyone who has chronic pain knows that occasionally, for no apparent reason, you will have a painful flare-up that will slow you down and aggravate some of your symptoms. Sometimes you over-do your exercise in the garden—you dig too deep or pull too hard, and this leaves your body sore due to unfamiliar repetitive motions. You can easily suffer injuries while lifting, moving, and carrying in the garden. Simply bending over can pull a back muscle, so be cautious. Listen to your body. If you feel weak or sore, slow down. Most importantly, ask for assistance in the garden when you need it.

If your flare-up or injury seems especially concerning, please consult with your health professional. Chances are, however, that the doctor will suggest you keep exercising regularly but change the pace to reduce stress on joints, back, and muscles. Abstaining from heavier aerobic activities might be a viable change that works, but reducing the level of intensity—slowing down your walking speed, for instance—can make a tremendous difference. Performing slow isometric exercises can sometimes help. Isometric exercises are typically performed by tensing a muscle in a contraction without physically moving the body part. Think about continuing stretching and isometric exercises that reduce quick motions and involve thoughtful, slower movement.

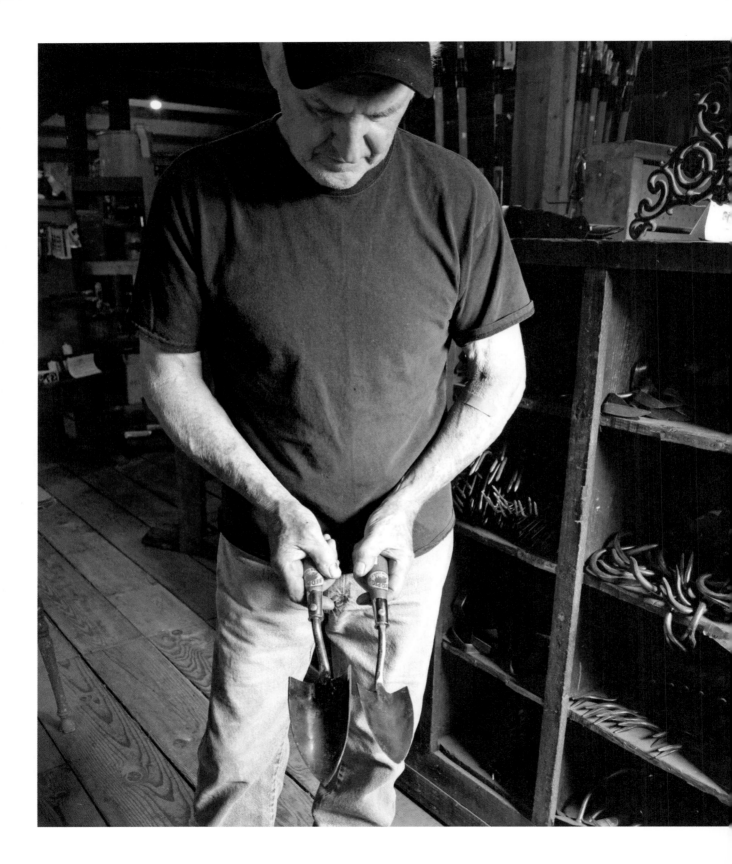

9

GARDEN TOOLS AND TECHNIQUES

ONE OF THE benefits of gardening, when considered as part of a workout program, is that it is an activity that combines multiple principles of exercise. Stretching, aerobic, and strengthening exercises all play a part. Your personal physical condition and your health professional's advice will dictate what level of activity will be most suited to your needs.

In 2012, it was reported that more than 86 million people in the United States are homeowners. Typical American yards are large and can be challenging to maintain. With this in mind, I have always found it interesting that the larger media world seems to refer to gardening as a "hobby." Many Americans see yard work such as mowing and weeding as a necessary weekly maintenance chore, not as a hobby. Making lawn maintenance and gardening a wellness choice—filled with fun, beauty, and health—is a positive way for homeowners to turn a chore into a transformational activity.

In addition, the Consumer Product Safety Commission (CPSC) states that emergency rooms treat more than 400,000 garden tool-related accidents each year. So, having an awareness of specific activities that might strain muscles and

OPPOSITE: Master blacksmith and toolmaker Bob Denman of Red Pig Tools advises using lightweight tools for short-handled tool chores and heavier tools for long-handled tool chores. He states that the heavier weight of a long-handled tool, for example, means your tools do more of the work for you. A short-handled tool that is heavy puts undo strain on your wrists and hands.

joints and of choosing and using the right tools can help you stay healthier and prevent accidents and injury.

VARY ACTIVITY TO PREVENT INJURY AND ACCIDENTS

One way to encourage wellness in the garden is to prevent injury by varying chores. Break garden activities into chunks that distribute and change up the type of movements you are making. For example, let's say that you have mowing, weeding, soil amending, and planting planned for a Saturday in early spring. It is your first time out in the garden after winter, so it's important to take it easy. Your body needs to acclimate.

Consider this: Try push-mowing a section of your yard, then take a break and weed a little along the garden beds. Mowing requires standing and walking movements, but weeding requires bending and stretching movements. They are different actions and switching between them regularly enables your body to stretch and modify positions

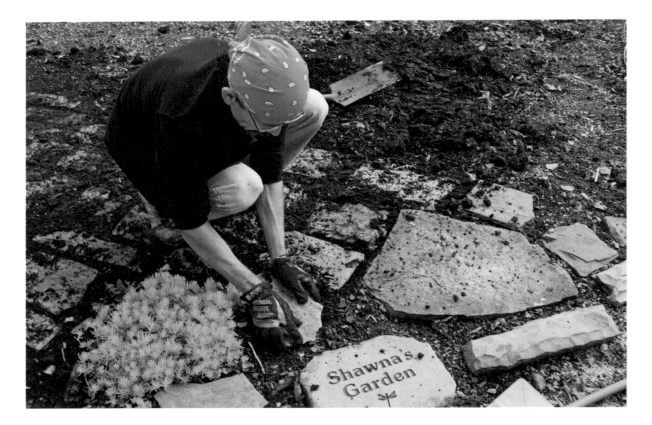

Vary activities while you are working in the garden and be sure to ask for help if needed. When my osteoarthritis is acting up, I ask friends and garden helpers like Jesús Martinez to work with me in the garden. It reduces physical strain on me and also motivates me to stay out in the fresh air as long as possible.

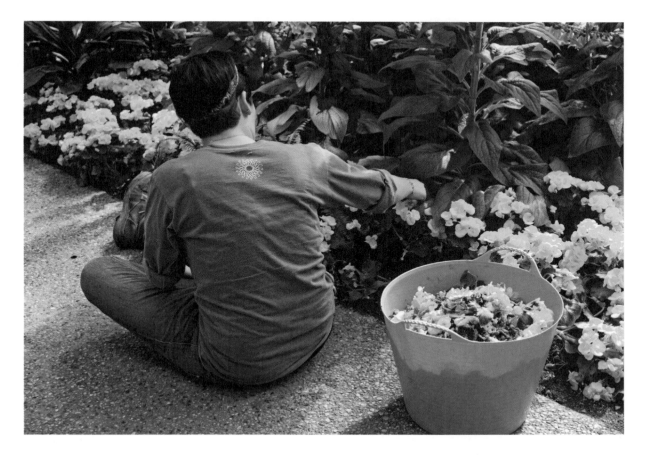

Instead of bending over at the waist, consider sitting down on the ground or with a short stool in order to weed or tend low-to-the-ground garden beds. It will help reduce back strain.

between exercise types, relieving stress. Take another break and add a few bags of soil to the beds. Then go back to mowing. Change activities again after you have pushed your mower for a while, and plant a few vegetables. This constant variation helps prevent your muscles and joints from getting locked into stiffness.

According to Dava Sobel and Arthur C. Klein, who wrote *Arthritis: What Exercises Work*, "Aim to maintain an awareness of your posture and movements as you work. This means keeping your back straight and bending with your knees when you must get down to ground level. Stay loose by occasionally shrugging and rolling your shoulders as you work. Carry flats or potted plants high and close to your body, so they don't force you to stoop over. For really heavy loads, use a wheelbarrow." I suggest using a more stable two-wheel wheelbarrow rather than a one-wheel wheelbarrow that can easily get out of balance.

HOW TO MOW CORRECTLY

Lawnmowers cause as many as 200,000 injuries and approximately 75 deaths per year, according to the US Consumer Product Safety Commission. Beyond the obvious dangers of blade-contact injuries, there are additional concerns of back and other muscle injuries caused by using push mowers.

Some push mowers also require a rip cord start-up. This involves bending and pulling, which can also strain ligaments, joints, and back muscle. Other common orthopedic injuries related to push lawnmower use include spinal injuries, shoulder dislocations, rotator cuff tears, and tendon injuries.

Before using a push mower or reel mower, be sure to ask for help to get the mower positioned in place if you need it. Do not lift a mower without assistance, and get help with starting the mower if you have a condition that will be aggravated by pulling the rip cord. Wear supportive shoes with arch support when mowing and consider wearing gloves to enhance your gripping ability. Be sure that the handles are placed in a position that allows you to stand straight; bending and pushing can easily injure your back. Take frequent breaks.

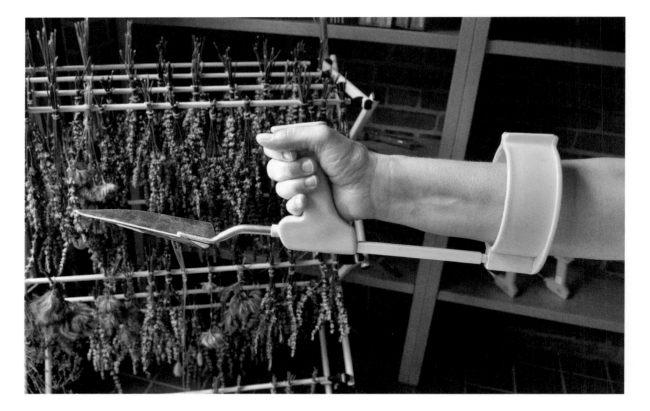

Shop for ergonomic tools that will work well for your particular health condition. Consult with your health professionals to better understand what part of your body might need relief and purchase tools with their guidance in mind.

GARDEN LIFTING

Sprains, pulls, and muscle pain can happen when lifting virtually anything in the garden. Soil and rotted manure often come in 50-pound bags. While it might be easy for you to toss a 50-pound bag over your shoulder, once it lands it can compress the spine, twist your shoulder, and hurt your back in a number of ways. First rule to follow: find a partner to help you lift heavy items. It can make a real difference.

Do not bend and lift: bending over and then lifting puts particular strain on your lower back. It forces your back to support the weight of the upper body as well as of the item you are lifting. Bending also moves the item you are lifting farther away from your body, creating additional problems with lower spine and causing muscle fatigue. Additionally, bending combined with twisting can cause intensive muscle and ligament strain.

Instead of risking injury, break a large or unwieldy load up into smaller parts so you can lift less weight at any one time. When lifting, it is important to bring the load in very close to your body, tighten your tummy muscles, and use your legs to power the load up. Keep your back straight during the lifting experience. Start from a squatting position. If extra support is needed, place one knee on the ground and one knee raised up before lifting. Go slow and be cautious: a fast lift can cause injury even when you are in a safe position.

Be sure to place the weight you are lifting somewhere between mid-thigh and your shoulder, do not boost it high up on your chest. Keep the load close to your body if you have to carry it any distance. Using common sense and a prevention mindset can significantly reduce injury or reduce chronic pain issues.

USE SHORT-HANDLED TOOLS WHEN POSSIBLE

While many people wait until they have pain and soreness before they seek an ergonomic solution, using properly designed tools at any stage of your physical health—whether you have an existing condition or not—will help keep you ahead of the injury game.

Do you have a physical limitation with your hands or arms? Then you might choose a short-handled trowel that addresses your condition. Ergonomic garden tools are specifically built to be easier on muscles and joints and so offer an opportunity for a gardener to actively participate in work he or she loves.

When seeking short-handled tools, look for lightweight tools that feel good in your hand and decrease strain when lifted. Pay attention to your pain-sensitivity zone. For instance, if you have chronic pain or another inflammatory issue in your wrists, focus on reducing strain in the wrist area by avoiding tools that force you to make strong twisting motions with your hands. Garden tools with a special curved handle that allow you to hold it in a "handshake" position cause significantly less strain than a straight-handled model. There are many styles of this handle on the market—curved handles, right-angled fist grips, T-grips, and wide-handled grips. Find one that works for you.

Digging techniques with short-handled tools should be done with lighter loads. Digging in a garden container with a trowel, for example,

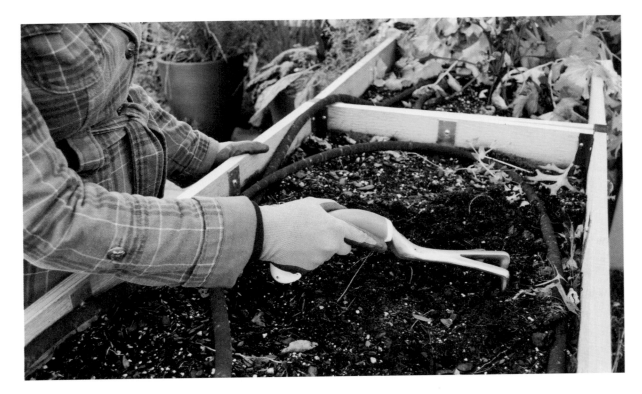

Effective short-handled tools that allow for a "handshake grip" on the curved handle include this Ergonomic Cultivator by Radius Garden. Whether you have a condition like arthritis or not, using more ergonomic tools will result in reduced strain and pain in the garden.

becomes easier if you use smaller strokes and less soil per trowel scoop. If lifting a scoop or trowel gives you an issue, try using a three-pronged cultivator, which functions as an extension of your fingers in its cultivating reach and enables you to dig without putting undo pressure on your fingers and wrist. This means your hands, arms, and back will be less strained.

Another way to manage short-handled tools if you have a weak grip or other issues is to wrap your tool handles with pipe insulation or a swimming pool noodle to widen your grip.

Pruners are extremely useful tools in the garden, but they can be hard on your body because they require repetitive movement that can be stressful on your back, arms, and hands. Using the right pruning tool with sharpened blades makes a tremendous difference in the ease of each cut. Make sure your cutting tools are the right size for your hand. Do not use dull pruners or a tool that forces your hand to twist, which puts pressure on joints. Choose ratchet pruners for tough jobs as the ratcheting mechanism will slice through thick branches with little effort.

If you have a weakened grip or problems pruning with traditional pruners, consider switching to small loppers that can be operated with two hands. Add your handy-dandy swimming pool noodle or pipe insulation to the loppers to widen the grip. Keep your cutting tools well-oiled so they are easier to use.

LONG-HANDLED TOOLS

Use the right tool for the right job. For example, when turning over heavy clay soil, it is often more effective to use a border fork or planting spade rather than a large shovel. This is because a large shovel offers more resistance than the narrow tines of a fork or a narrow spade.

Like the short-handled gardening tools, there are various ergonomic shapes and designs available for long-handled tools, including a completely round grip, T-handle, or extended grip handle. Sliding a swimming pool noodle or pipe insulation over the handle can help widen the grip area for the long-handled tool. Secure it with duct tape.

While it is much better to use a lightweight tool for your short-handled efforts, it's usually best to use a heavier tool for heavier projects. Heavier long-handled tools do more of the work for you—heavier shovels, forks, cultivators, spades, and hoes drop easily into heavy soil, enabling you to pull, push, or dig with less strain and using the weight of the tool in your favor.

Instead of bending forward in an awkward "reach and pull" movement with a long-handled tool, bring the tool close to you whenever possible. If using a shovel or fork, stand very close to the tool as you are using it. Step firmly on the top of

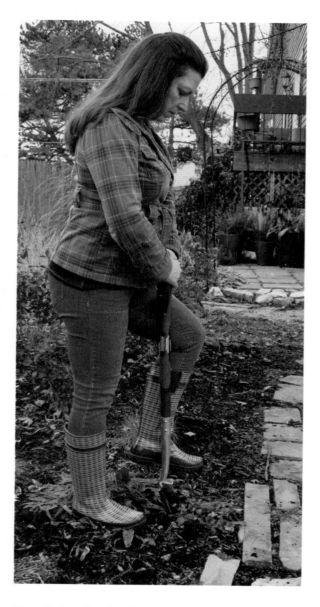

When digging with a shovel or a tool like this PRO Stainless Weeder by Radius Garden, be sure to place your body immediately over the digging area as I have in the photo, with the shovel or digging tool directly at your feet. Digging becomes easier on your back when you keep your tools close to your body. If you overextend your arms and back while digging, it can cause back, neck, and arm pain.

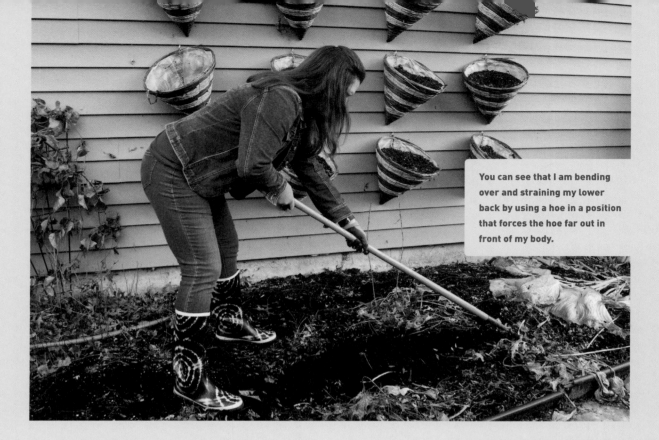

You can see that I am bending over and straining my lower back by using a hoe in a position that forces the hoe far out in front of my body.

THE BROOM SWEEP TECHNIQUE

The "broom sweep technique" is a healthier way to use a long-handled tool such as a hoe.

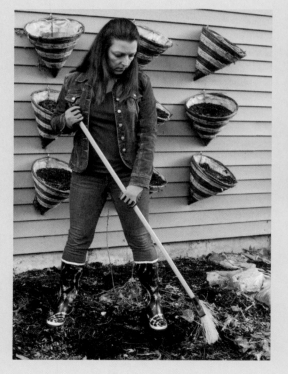

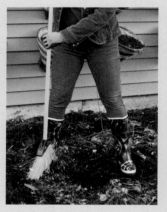

RIGHT: Notice how I have a broom in illustration of a long-handled garden tool. With the tool placed in the soil, use the same motions for digging as you would for sweeping with a broom. Move from left to right without lifting the tool out of the soil. This reduces strain on your back.

ABOVE: You can see how the broom does not get extended past my right foot. This "broom sweep technique" enables you to hold your long-handled garden tool more closely to your body, which can help prevent lower back injuries. You will also have a better grip on your tool.

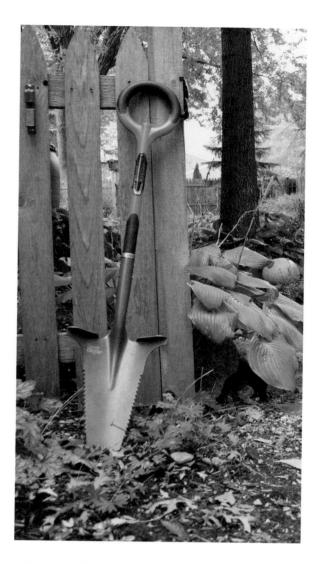

the shovel, letting your legs push the tool into the soil in order to reduce strain on your back and joints. Do not twist and dump. Instead, move your feet and turn your entire body to move the soil, compost, or gravel you are working with.

When using long-handled tools and bending over a job, we gardeners have a tendency to look up, periscoping the neck by pulling the chin up and away from the chest, during the digging process. This puts all the strain of the dig on the upper back and neck. Physical therapists recommend "keeping your eye on the ball." Put your head and neck in a position where you are looking directly at your project and don't move your neck in unusual or uncomfortable positions during the garden project.

Using tools that have a wide or ergonomically shaped handle enables people with gripping conditions to more easily manipulate the tools in the garden. The Root Slayer from Radius Garden has a round, ergonomically designed handle that makes it easier to hold.

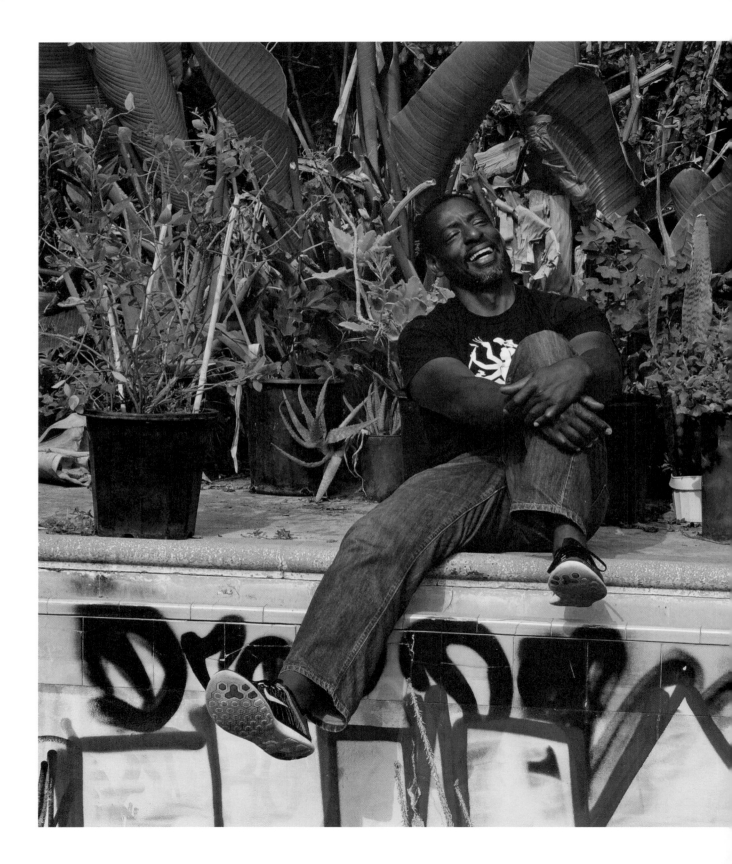

𝟣𝟢

GARDEN IN A FOOD DESERT

RON FINLEY IS a Los Angeles–based gardener. He credits a gardening lifestyle—healthy eating and organic gardening—as the primary ingredient for his wellness. He lives in South Central Los Angeles, an urban area in southern California filled with baking cement, liquor stores, fast-food restaurants, and very few grocery stores. As urban areas go, this part of the city is definitively a food desert.

Food deserts are primarily defined as areas within urban communities where the local community has no access to fresh produce within walking distance. There is plenty of fast food, but in order to find fresh whole food, the residents must leave their immediate community. Grocery stores can be 5 to 10 miles away from city neighborhoods, and impoverished residents without cars must pay a bus or taxi to take them to another area to find food. This is more than an inconvenience for thousands of people who live below the poverty level because it becomes a hardship to find healthy food. Moving away from the area might not be a choice for these people because of housing affordability. Ron recognized all of these difficulties and decided to bring fresh food back into the neighborhoods.

OPPOSITE: Ron Finley, seen here on the side of his swimming pool plant nursery near South Central Los Angeles, is making a difference with his team of volunteers from the Ron Finley Project, a not-for-profit foundation that teaches gardening by building more gardens around South Central Los Angeles and the Los Angeles community.

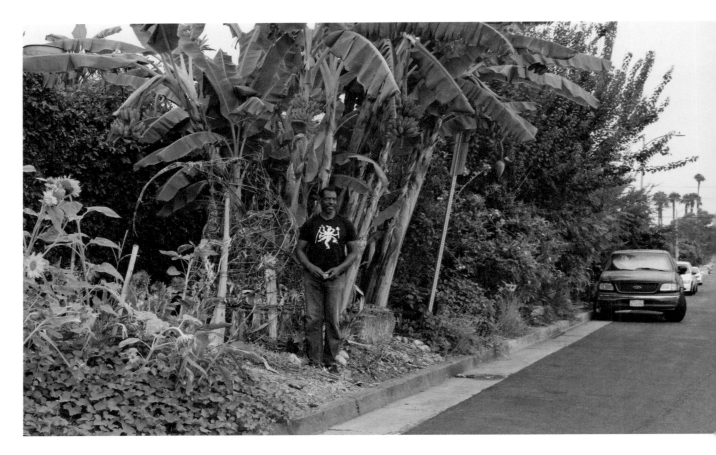

Ron Finley gardens in his "hell strip," the area between the street and the sidewalk. In most major cities, homeowners are required to maintain this grassy strip, but it is considered illegal to grow other plants, shrubs, trees, or vegetables here. Check your local city ordinances before planting in your hell strip. If there are strict rules against it, consider contacting local city management to see how you might be able to change the rules with the city's approval.

According to an article published by the United States Department of Agriculture titled, "Access to Affordable Nutritious Food: Measuring and Understanding Food Deserts and Their Consequences," 23.5 million people live in areas that are more than 1 mile from a large supermarket. To be considered a "low-access community," a minimum of 500 people or 33 percent of the census tract's population must live farther than 1 mile from a supermarket or large grocery store. For rural census tracts, the distance is more than 10 miles.

Ron's research into food deserts began when he realized that his own neighborhood was devoid of a grocery store within walking distance, yet was filled with fast-food restaurants and gas stations that offered only higher priced items with much lower nutritional values. Large supermarkets were unwilling to invest in the area because the low incomes of many of the local citizens, combined with the higher crime rate of surrounding neighborhoods. Growing a garden brought fresh flavor, vitamins, and health to citizens' dinner plates and soon became a healthy solution for Ron and his local community.

RECLAIMING THE HELL STRIP

Although Ron saw the unkempt, grassy, unused hell strip area in front of his home as "his" to grow on, mostly because he had to mow and maintain it regularly, the City of Los Angeles saw it as right-of-way property owned by the city. Ron was taken to court and has since continued to fight for his island garden. He eventually got the rules for hell strips changed throughout the Los Angeles area.

Concerned not only about the food desert hardship for his community but also a modern societal trend toward inactivity and indoor living, Ron Finley brought his community together and began growing, harvesting, and sharing from his home garden. He envisions a community where kids understand their nutritional needs and where communities embrace the gardening, learning about and sharing the best of the earth's fresh-grown food.

Planting a hell-strip garden is a perfect way to help dissipate the heat-island effect that plagues major cities. These additional plantings interrupt large areas of pavement help reduce the temperature of surrounding air and ground space. Encouraging people to grow their own food saves significant money and can offer neighbors a source of income as well: once you grow the food, you can choose to consume it or sell it to the community. Even better, getting outside and planting with

neighbors keeps people away from their televisions and engages them with physical and emotional healing, putting them in touch with the soil while helping others in their community. It is Ron's heart and soul belief that gardening everywhere you can, whenever you can, builds wellness.

Gorgeous potato vines stretch along the front of Ron's street garden. There are tropical plants of all sorts mixed in with herbs such as basil and sage. He grows figs in the small space along with every kind of vegetable imaginable. As you walk along the sidewalk, banana trees arch over your head, and coolness awaits you beneath their shade on a 100-degree, sweltering Los Angeles day. The scent of fresh herbs waft through the air. Ron is in his element when he stands in his gardens: he encourages neighbors to pick fruits and vegetables as they need

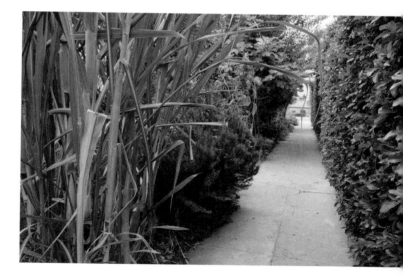

Ron grows figs, pomegranates, potatoes, sunflowers, herbs, and vegetables of all kinds in this garden area in between the sidewalk and street. He shares the food with his friends and neighbors to help make a difference in the food desert community where he lives.

to. His efforts have resulted in thousands of people in the community growing their own food for the wellness and health of their community.

Eventually, Ron coalesced his many efforts into the Ron Finley Project, a not-for-profit foundation that enables an energetic group of employees and volunteers to expand their planting and educational initiatives by building more gardens around South Central Los Angeles and the Los Angeles community at large.

PLANTS IN THE SWIMMING POOL

After Ron planted his hell strip, it soon became clear to him that every square inch of his property should also be a growing space for plants, herbs, vegetables, and bees. His efforts have produced a uniquely creative and beautiful garden filled with life and art. More importantly, he firmly contributes his fitness level to consistent work in the garden: it is his inspiration and passion.

At the back of his property, confined within a fence made of cement bricks, is an abandoned swimming pool. Having long since lost the ability to operate as a pool, the structure is instead filled with Ron's immense plant nursery. There is purposeful graffiti painted over the walls of the pool, but more than half of the bottom the pool is full of plants of every kind.

When I asked Ron about why the pool was gardened in this fashion his reply was simple: "It was empty and needed to feed people." Indeed.

Ron Finley's astounding graffiti- and plant-filled swimming pool at his South Los Angeles home shows how to reuse and recycle. While the broken-down pool might not have been useful or affordable for him to maintain, converting it to a plant nursery became an important part of his growing efforts.

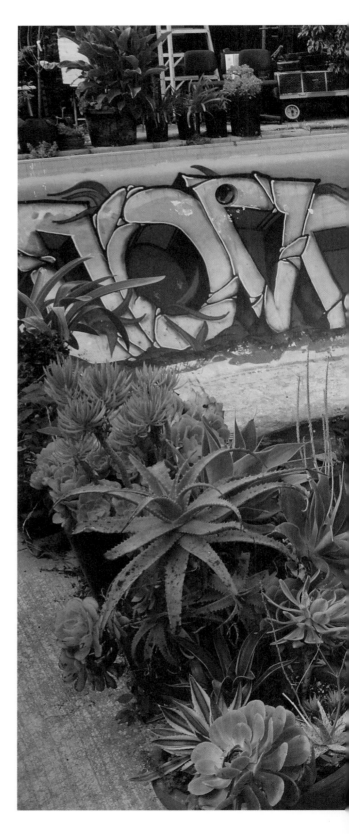

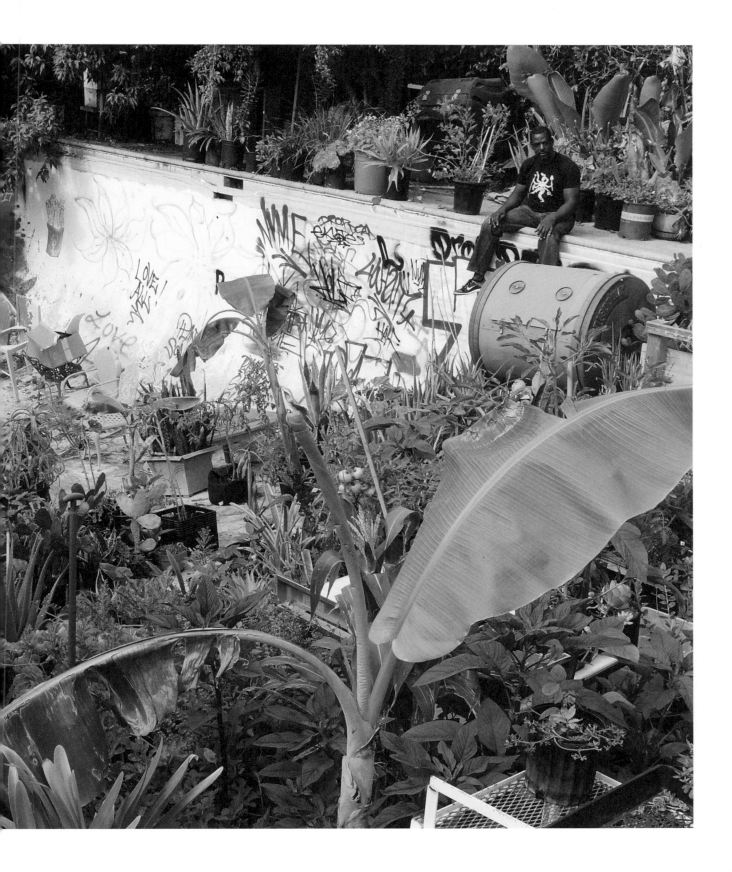

Tips to Prevent Food Waste

- Plan meals in advance to avoid impulse buys. Go to the grocery or farmers market with a specific list and buy exactly what you need.
- Help your community by buying the ugly fruit and vegetables that usually gets thrown out at the grocer, even though it tastes just as good as the perfect produce.
- Label, package, and freeze your fresh food in order to extend its life. Canning or pickling is also a great solution.
- Use the "first in, first out principle," or "FIFO." As you unpack your groceries, move the older products to the front of the refrigerator instead of pushing it to the back.
- Consume leftovers or share them with friends in your community.
- Choose the day before shopping day as a "use what we have" meal and use up all your leftovers and food in your cabinets.
- Donate your extra fruits, vegetables, and canned goods to a local food pantry, particularly if you live in a food desert.
- Have meat scraps and bits and pieces of onion or potato skins? Mix them together in a large stock pot with water and make broth before you toss them out.
- Compost all your fruit and vegetable scraps.
- Contact your elected officials and ask them to support legislation that will help reduce food waste.

I would agree—wherever you have a spare inch, you should incorporate plants as an active solution for your own health and the health of others. Why not incorporate plants to feed yourself and your community and truly make a difference?

FOOD WASTE

With all the concern for people living in food deserts, we also have a devastating amount of food loss. The World Resources Institute (WRI) suggests that, in 2013, global food loss and waste totaled up to 24 percent of all the food calories produced, or one in four calories, worth approximately $1 trillion. According to the WRI, "Food loss and waste have many negative economic and environmental impacts. Economically, they represent a wasted investment that can reduce farmers' incomes and increase consumers'

expenses. . . . We estimate that if the current rate of food loss and waste were cut in half (from 24 percent to 12 percent) by the year 2050, the world would need about 1,314 trillion kilocalories (kcal) less food per year. . . . That savings—1,314 trillion kcal—is roughly 22 percent of the 6,000 trillion kcal per year gap between food available today and that needed in 2050. Thus, reducing food loss and waste could be one of the leading global strategies for achieving a sustainable food future."

Additionally, there is an extremely high environmental cost globally: organic food waste is the second highest landfill ingredient worldwide and is the largest source of methane emissions. This means that humans are causing unnecessary greenhouse gas emissions simply by wasting food. Landfills around the world are overfilled and are running out of space for all our waste.

HELPING FEED YOUR NEIGHBORHOOD

According to the Garden Writers Association (GWA) Foundation, "Since 1995, over 20 million pounds of produce providing over 80 million meals have been donated by American gardeners. All of this has been achieved without government subsidy or bureaucratic red tape—just people helping people." The GWA Foundation created a Plant a Row for the Hungry public service program to encourage communities to help feed hungry Americans. Knowing that there are 84 million households with a yard or garden in the United States, it makes sense to have every gardener plant one extra row.

Sharing food can start within your own neighborhood. Perhaps you live in a food desert region? Or perhaps you just have a balcony that is filled with vegetables? Either way, begin sharing your food: meet your neighbors and get to know them. You will soon discover who needs an extra cucumber or squash. Connecting with your neighbors is more than simply being friendly, it is also a strong step toward wellness. Social activities that promote emotional connections are good for mental health and contribute to your overall emotional fitness. Being well is a combination of meeting nutritional, physical, and emotional needs. Let your garden bring your neighbors when you share fresh herbs and vegetables.

Contact your local food pantries and find out if they will accept fresh food from the garden. Then deliver the fresh produce on their specific donation days so that food pantry patrons will

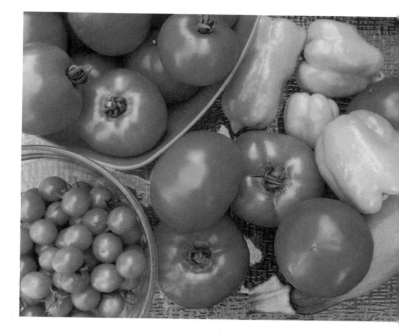

Growing food for your community is not the only thing to consider in regard to feeding people. Food waste is a $1 trillion global problem. Growing food and donating it where it will be put to good use is absolutely critical.

get the freshest and most nutritious vegetables possible. It is important to note that hundreds of hungry families are refused at food banks each year due to low staffing and resource availability. This means that it is more important than ever for you to meet your neighbors, learn what your community's needs are, and plant an extra row to connect people to a healthy organic meal whenever possible. This is about you and your health, but also the health of your neighbors. By keeping your community healthy, you are truly making a difference.

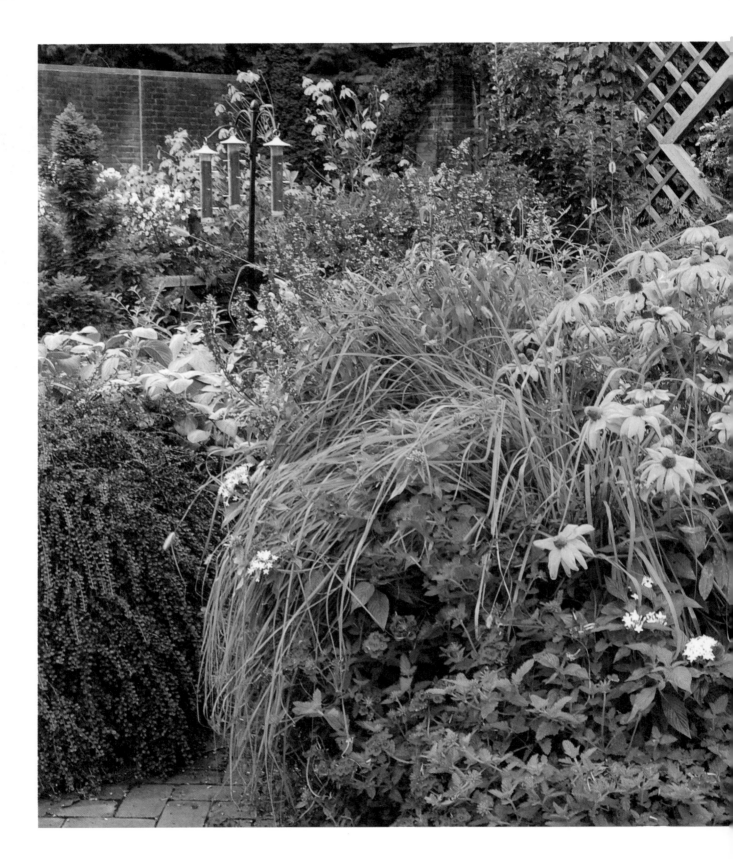

PART III

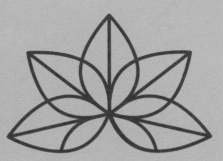

THERAPEUTIC GARDENING

Therapeutic gardens can be much like the Beuhler Enabling Garden at the Chicago Botanic Garden. Elevated beds make gardening physically easier if you have a specific health condition, but a therapeutic garden can also address your psychological, spiritual, and social needs.

Photo taken at Chicago Botanic Garden.

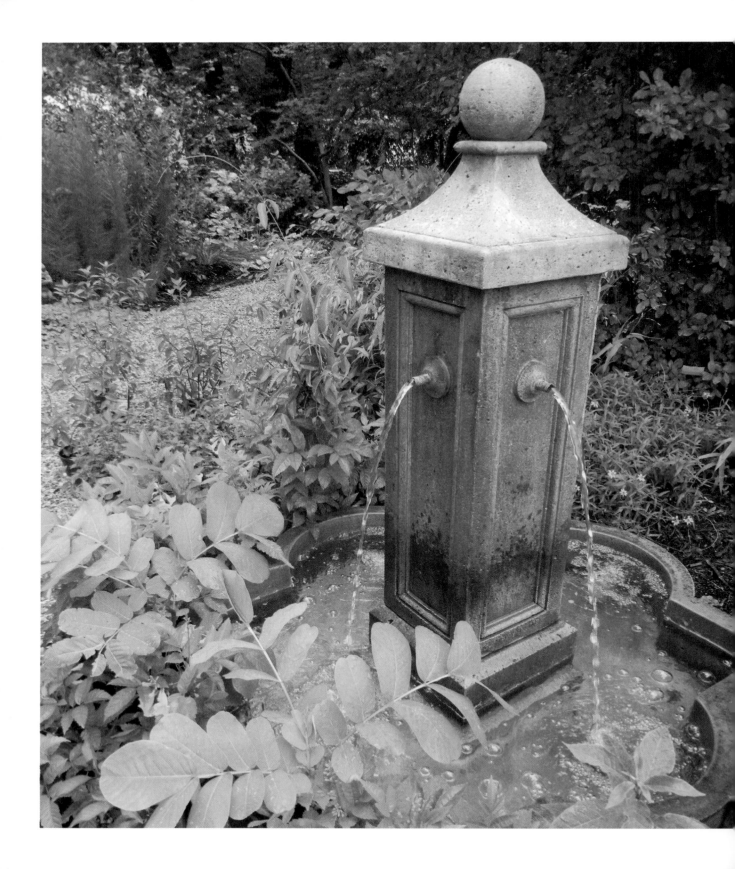

11

REDUCING ANXIETY AND DEPRESSION WITH GREEN ACTIVITIES

A THERAPEUTIC GARDEN is defined as a space where you can accomplish gardening and green activities that specifically address a person's psychological, spiritual, physical, and social needs. Therapeutic gardening can be far more than a traditional garden space: it can be expanded to include many outdoor landscaped areas, green spaces, and even activities that can be accomplished in a garden or open park expanse. Discovering an outdoor place where you can connect with nature therapeutically while performing green activities can be life changing. These "green activities" could be as specific as gardening, walking, running, or cycling in nature and garden-like locations, or they can be more widely interpreted in environmental conservation work.

BRAIN NEUROTRANSMITTERS IN THE GARDEN

While we know that the bacterium strain *Mycobacterium vaccae* has been shown to trigger the release of serotonin when a person has direct skin-to-soil contact, there is also further proof that dopamine levels increase in the brain when we participate in green activities.

Both serotonin and dopamine are pleasure-center neurotransmitters that are associated

OPPOSITE: Building gardens that connect visitors to nature might include water features that enhance an outdoor immersion in nature.

with happiness, pleasure, and love. Serotonin specifically regulates mood, memory, and impulse. Dopamine is closely tied to euphoria, enjoyment, and motivation. Dopamine is also responsible for those magical feelings of "falling in love." When depression is caused by a chemical imbalance, it is often associated with an insufficient level of dopamine in the brain.

SUNLIGHT AND SEROTONIN

Another proven serotonin stimulator is sunlight. By exercising outdoors in the garden or walking outdoors daily, you are exposing yourself to the daylight spectrum. It is a good practice to expose yourself to daylight without sunglasses for 20 minutes every day.

Dr. David Edelberg, MD, confirms in his book, *The Triple Whammy Cure*, that improving serotonin levels can reduce stress levels. The book, although applicable to most people, focuses on women's health. Dr. Edelberg states that the more serotonin you have, the better you are able to tolerate all types of extreme stress. He also proposes that women have less serotonin than men do, which makes them more susceptible to stress-related

Research over the last decade at universities from around the globe show that participation in a regular outdoor exercise can often be as effective as antidepressants in treating mild depression. One particular 16-week study done by the Department of Psychiatry and Behavioral Sciences at Duke University Medical Center in Durham, North Carolina, shows that the effects of exercise training on patients with major depression was as effective as taking anti-depressant medication. This means that aerobic movement that occurs while working in the garden and walking in the fresh air can be both physically and mentally restorative. *Photo taken at Longwood Gardens in Kennett Square, PA.*

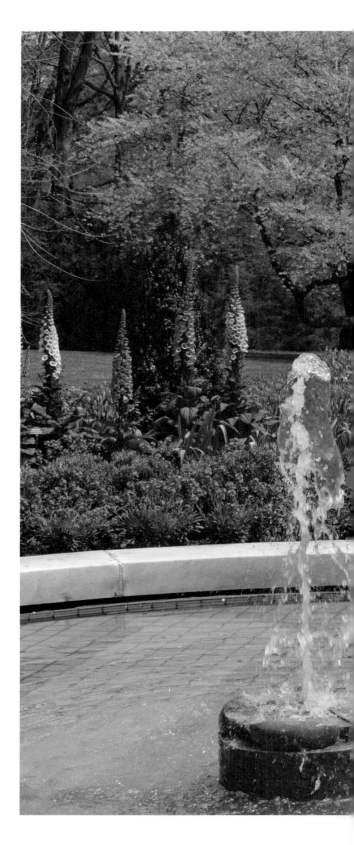

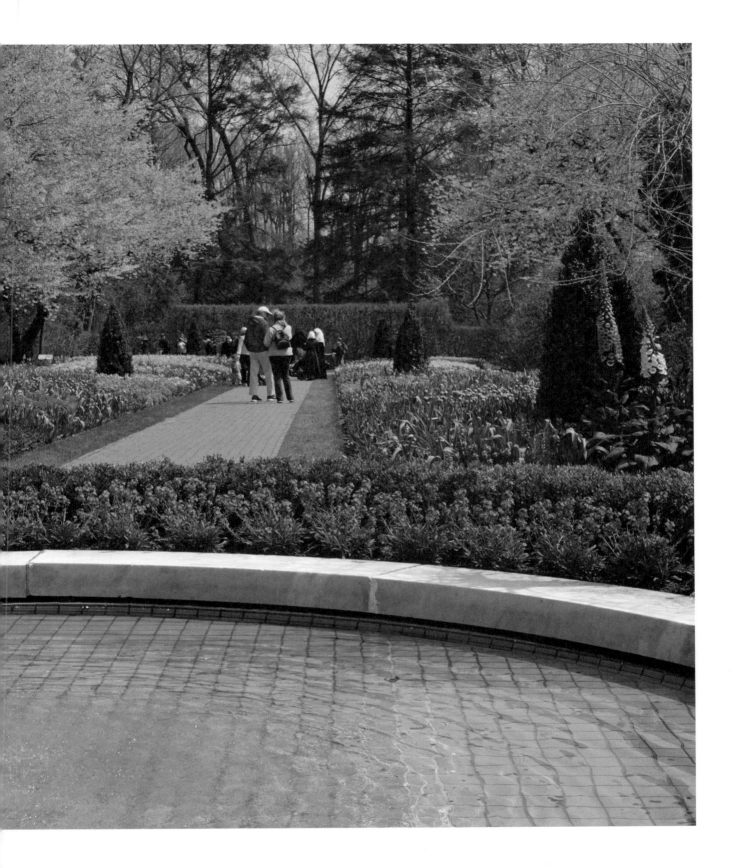

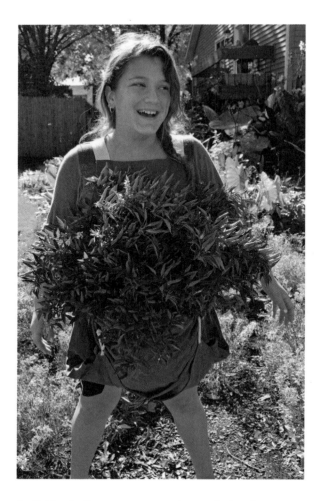

Sunlight and soil exposure are amazing serotonin enhancers. Getting out in the garden as a family, planting and harvesting vegetables, and getting in touch with nature can, in turn, give you a wonderful mood boost.

starting as the daylight ebbs in fall and stretching through the season until there is more daylight exposure after winter. SAD saps energy and can make you feel moody and sorrowful. Performing green activities outdoors with regular exposure to daylight has a significantly positive effect on the patient.

There are certain eye conditions, such as macular degeneration, that worsen with exposure to sunlight. If you suspect you have this condition or something similar, please contact your doctor for his advice before spending more time in the sunlight. Also, it is very important to wear sunscreen while working outdoors. This is critical even on cloudy days as the sun's rays are powerful and can easily overwhelm precious skin when least expected.

GREEN ACTIVITIES AND ENGAGING WITH NATURE

According to the Centers for Disease Control and Prevention statistical website, data from the National Health and Nutrition Examination Surveys from 2005 to 2008 show that antidepressant use has increased significantly: "About 1 in 10 Americans aged 12 and over takes anti-depressant medication." While there is no doubt that the stigma related to mental illness issues is dissipating, which encourages proper medication when necessary, it becomes critical to learn new ways to reduce pharmaceutical dependency whenever possible. It is possible to reduce anxiety, depression, and related medication use by increasing green activities, enabling people to find an alternative path to their personal wellness lifestyle.

issues in general. He encourages everyone to try daily sunlight exposure.

Sunlight exposure also appears to be an effective treatment for winter-based seasonal affective disorder (SAD). This particular type of depression is related to changes in the seasons,

"Mind" is an organization in the United Kingdom that assists millions of people online to learn how to cope with anxiety, depression, and other mental health issues. Mind also provides support directly through local chapters and conducts treatment studies through the University of Essex.

In one such report, "Ecotherapy—the Green Agenda for Mental Health," 94 percent of test subjects commented that they felt green exercise had furthered their mental health in a positive way. Additionally, the study stated that participants felt their physical health improved with outdoor walking. Respondents also reported decreased levels of depression and felt less fatigued and tense after walking outside, with increased mood and self-esteem.

In other words, outdoor activities such as gardening and walking can significantly influence your state of mind by triggering dopamine and serotonin levels and by connecting a person's very soul to the natural outdoor environment.

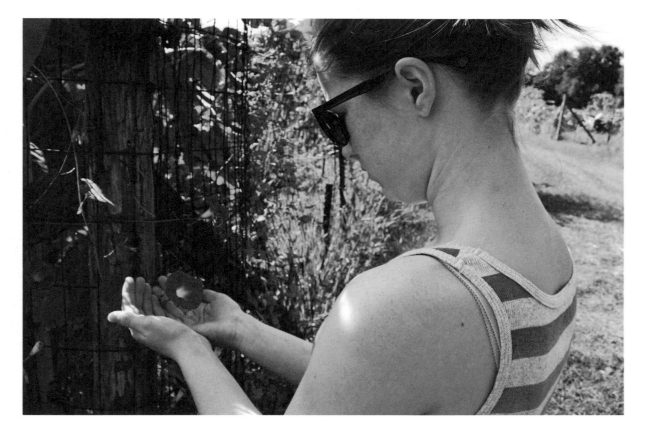

Connecting at an intimate level with your environment can stimulate positive hormones and reduce depression. Touch a morning glory or smell the soil. Stop to admire to plants, animals, and views you discover so that your brain can make a personal connection to the outdoor environment.

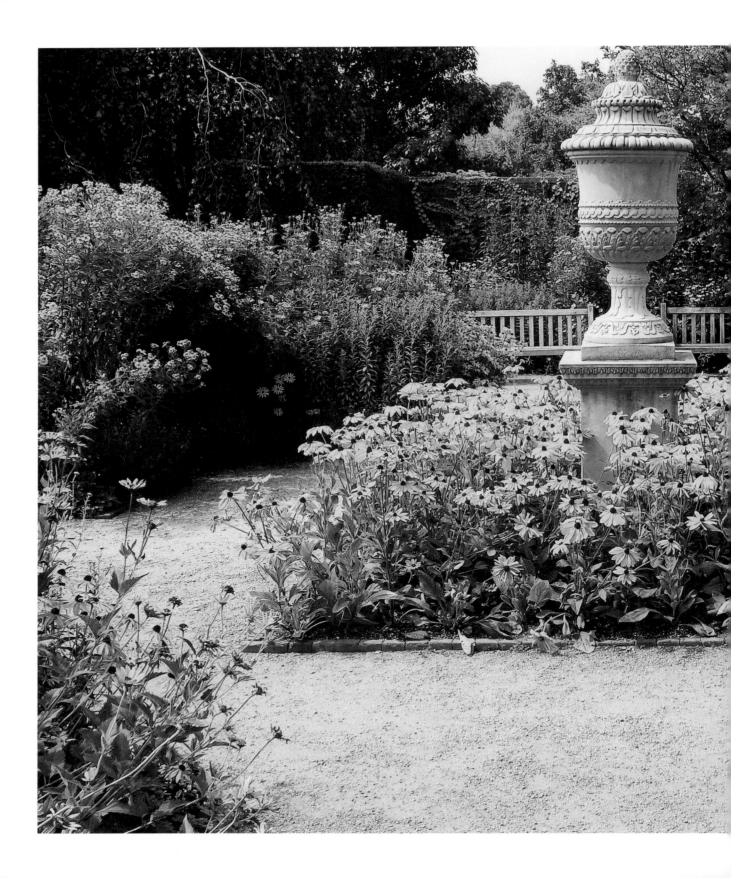

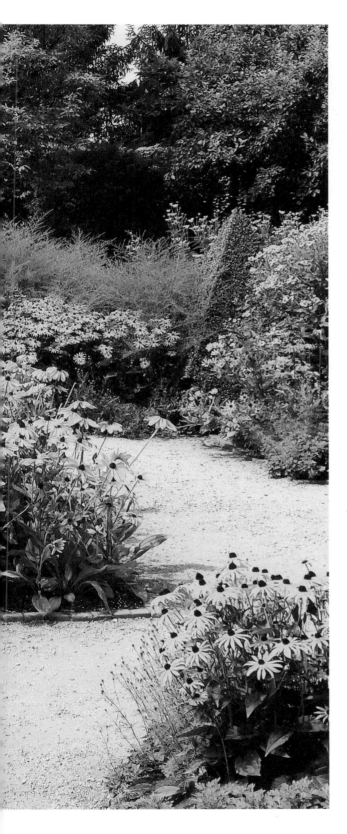

LIVING MINDFULLY

One of the great benefits of the garden and nature in general is that it lends itself to mindfulness. When your mind is filled with thoughts about work, finances, and family, there is no better cure than to weed or tend to your plants. Gardening causes our minds to be intrinsically focused on the present. Life's difficulties and dramas melt away as we address our task.

Plants need love. Tending them takes our eyes, our hands, and our hearts. In the garden, we hear the birds, the wind in the trees, the beauty and color in flowers. We touch the soil and plants, we smell the magnificence of all of nature on a spring day, we can taste the harvest of a strawberry. Gardening stimulates all the senses and the act of gardening is giving to someone else more important than ourselves: Mother Earth.

Living mindfully is often defined as "living in the moment." Without a doubt, organic gardening creates an environment where one must live in the present moment. Most importantly, the singular activity of gardening can calm an anxious mind and allow that focus to wash over you in a way very few things can.

An additional benefit of mindfulness is that the rhythmic tasks in the garden often set your thoughts to wander. Weeding and digging can stimulate your mind to drift through difficult

Treating memory loss and depression with daily gardening, growing plants familiar to patients, can make a tremendous difference. Growing plants with familiar scents, colors, and designs can stimulate memory. This monochromatic English garden design was created at the Chicago Botanic Garden.
Photo taken at Chicago Botanic Garden.

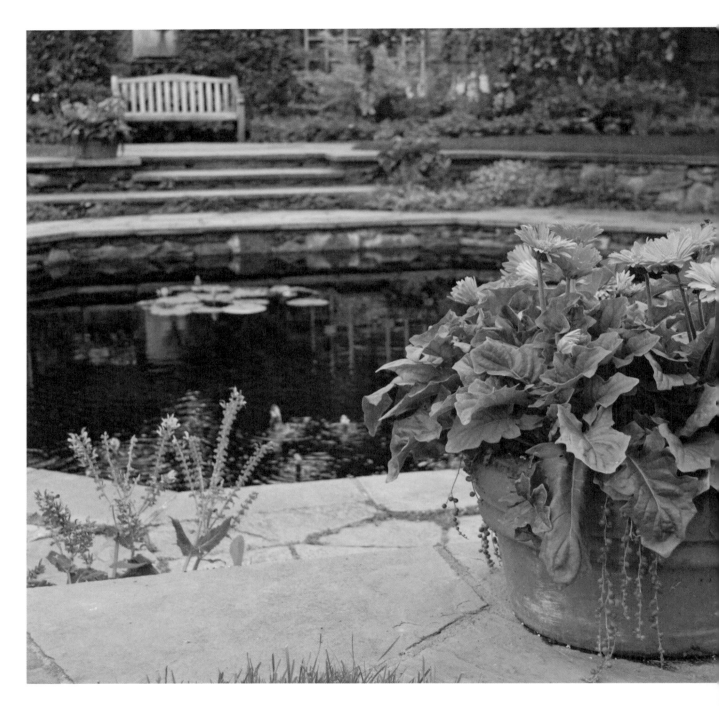

Living mindfully means engaging in the moment. When we rush through life without thought, we often miss important details. Having a garden area with a quiet seating area customized to the needs of those coming to the garden means visitors will be able to sit and observe the garden in a mindful way. *Photo taken at Chicago Botanic Garden.*

CHAPTER 11

problems our brain is trying to solve and can sometimes trigger a mental release to the block we had while staring blindly at the computer only minutes before.

MEMORY LOSS AND DEPRESSION

Living mindfully can become difficult when we have memory loss issues. Particularly prevalent amongst depression sufferers, short-term memory loss or brain-fog episodes can be particularly challenging. Other conditions such as Alzheimer's and dementia are also often associated with depressive moods caused by an inability to remember or perform recent activities related to short-term memory. Watching a friend or family member suffer through a memory disorder can be heartbreaking, but gardening and horticultural therapy can definitely help someone live a fuller lifestyle.

While short-term memory and brain-fog episodes can happen at any age, daily horticultural therapy can make a difference particularly in the elderly with depression and dementia. Horticultural therapy and exposure to gardens has been shown to be effective for improving sleep, agitation, and cognition in dementia patients. As a cognitive therapy, horticultural therapy can help someone learn new skills and regain their lost skills by helping to rebuild brain pathways. Overall, horticultural therapy is a healing method to improve memory and social interaction with limited adversative side effects. Improving stress levels, feelings of well-being and self-esteem is also possible with horticultural therapy.

While there is no instant cure for clinically diagnosed depression, there are ways to utilize a garden to make a difference. Often people who have conditions that affect short-term memory still have an intimate connection with their long-term memory. For instance, many Alzheimer patients can remember music and television shows from their childhood. When listening to songs from their childhood, faces will go from slack to excited, and the patients will sometimes sing along to the music word-for-word. With this in mind, try building a special garden focused on long-term memories for the people who have memory challenges that might help engage positive memories. Recreate plants, flowers, patio furniture, and outdoor living experiences that trigger the five senses with historic and memorable scents, sounds, and scenes for the patient or garden visitor. This stimulation of long-term memory triggers—such as smelling roses from a childhood rose garden—can help open up cognitive thoughts.

A 2011 multi-study review, "Environmental Science & Technology," learned that compared to being indoors, performing green activity exercises outdoors in natural environments worked strongly to build more positive mental states among study subjects. They felt reenergized with less depression, anger, and confusion.

But even if you do not suffer from depression, anxiety, or memory loss, you should incorporate these activities into your wellness lifestyle. Making a difference for ourselves emotionally is as important as our physical care, and with your medical professional's guidance, a garden can change our mindset for the positive.

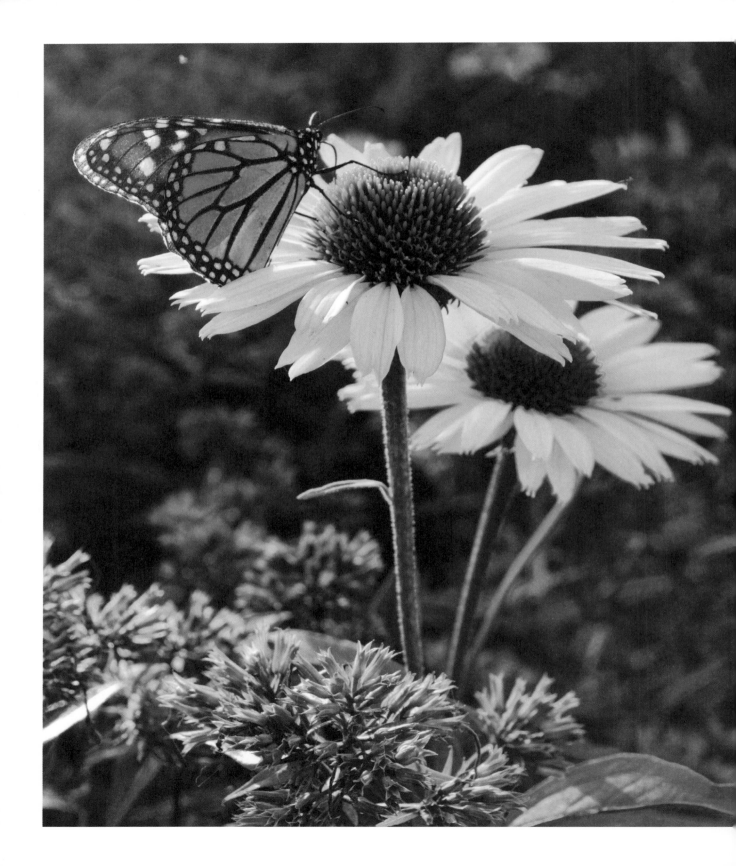

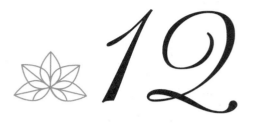

THERAPEUTIC GARDEN
DESIGN SOLUTIONS

THIS SECTION OF *The Wellness Garden* is a quick tip guide to get you thinking about potential healing garden design ideas. It is not a manual on evidence-based design (EBD), which is the use of quantitative scientific research to design environments that facilitate activities meant to specifically improve outcomes for health and wellness. Just as there is no replacement for consulting a physician to diagnose your physical ailments, there is also no replacement for a formally educated EBD expert, who can definitely connect you to a garden designed with your very specific medical and health needs. Should you want more formal guidance with EBD, see the Therapeutic Landscapes Network website at www.healinglandscapes.org to find formally certified therapeutic designers, consultants, guidelines, and additional resources.

OPPOSITE: While therapeutic gardens are primarily built to help humans with mental and physical health issues, they can also present a unique opportunity to connect with pollinators, birds, and other animals. An organic pollinator garden, for example, attracts pollinators that support the environment and also visually stimulates the observer.

DEFINING YOUR HEALING OR WELLNESS LIFESTYLE GARDEN

Large healing gardens are most likely to be found in settings that encompass health care facilities: mental health hospitals, Alzheimer's treatment facilities, cancer treatment centers, nursing homes, and other like institutions. Therapeutic and healing garden designs are all about structuring a garden so that it helps you live your own wellness lifestyle and make you feel better, healthier, and more content. You do not have to be ill or in pain to discover the benefits of a therapeutic garden. You need merely step into the garden to feel its effects.

While a large or commercial therapeutic garden at a facility might be formally designed and structured by horticultural therapy design professionals, it is definitely possible for you to assemble your own less formal design for your patio, walls, or balcony using a little common sense and intuition. Keep in mind that you can always reach out to an EBD professional if you need more advice.

WHERE TO GET STARTED

When designing a healing or therapeutic garden for your wellness lifestyle, the first thought is to make a long list of many items to incorporate. This can create a cluttered and confusing area. Instead, focus on keeping the garden very simple so that it is easy to traverse, has an understandable and effective wellness principle, and shows a unified design.

In Martha M. Tyson's therapeutic garden design book *The Healing Landscape; Therapeutic Outdoor Environments*, she writes that the initial objective of designing a therapeutic garden is

Healing gardens can also be "landscapes," much like this gorgeous view. Therapeutic landscaping offers beautiful vistas and other techniques that address a person's unique mental and physical health issues. *Photo taken at Chicago Botanic Garden.*

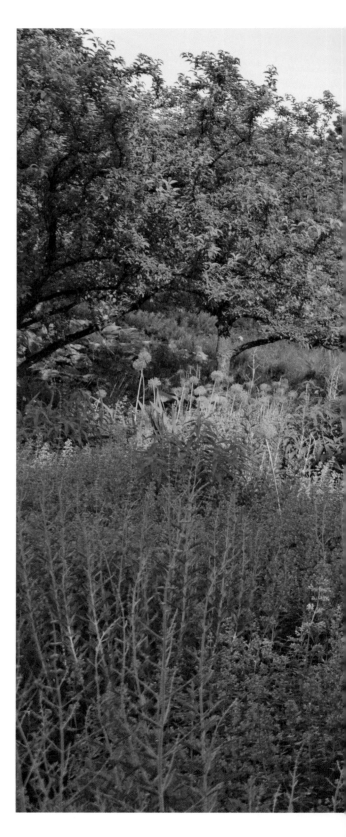

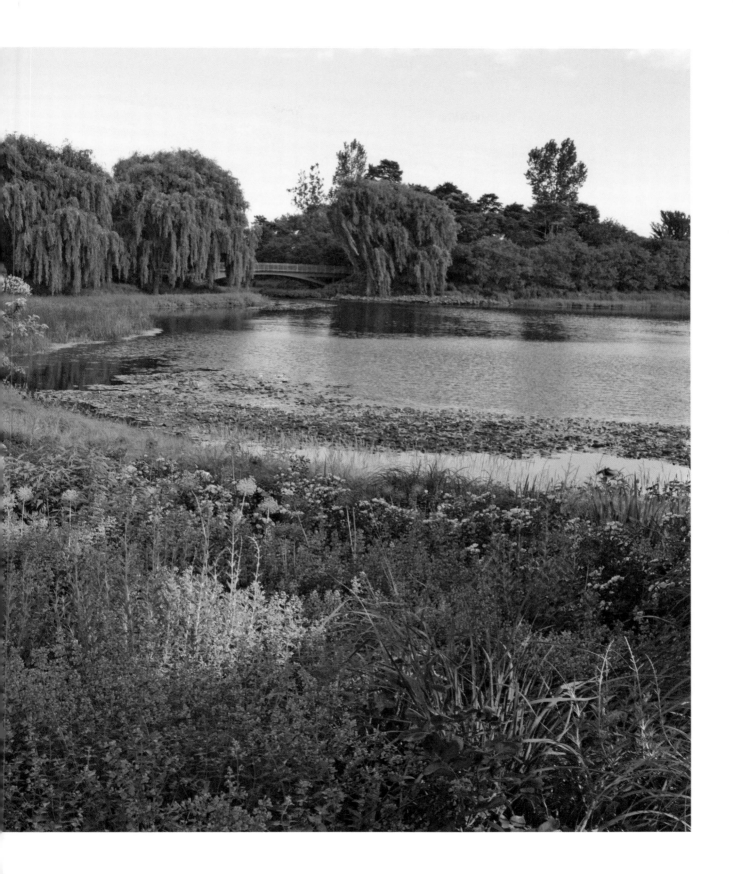

Five Tips for a Healing Garden Design

1. **Use fewer chemicals.** Having a garden that is organic is important so that it is environmentally friendly. Use natural materials in your garden area that will promote health and are safe for the environment. Materials like pots or edging should not be treated with chemicals. This attentiveness to safety in a garden area where people will be touching, smelling, and consuming plants is critical for wellness.

2. **Conserve water.** While it is acceptable to plant a garden that might be a water waster, it makes sense for ease of maintenance and the environment to build a garden that has lower water requirements. Use a drip system, and place plants with similar water requirements together.

3. **Functionality is key.** Your garden should address specific healing needs and accommodate and support any limitations gardeners or garden visitors might have. While having a beautiful or visually pleasing garden is important, make sure that your garden design is functional. For example, provide wide and open pathways, have plants that address the specific needs of the garden visitor, and make sure the garden is safe for visitors and gardeners.

4. **Keep it easy to manage.** Having an elaborate or difficult to maintain garden will countermand your basic need to have a garden that is enjoyable. Create a garden design that is easy to look after and sustain.

5. **Be money-wise.** Plot your expenses for the garden to keep your design cost-effective. With smart planning you can reduce, reuse, and recycle garden art, pathway material, and garden furniture to keep costs down. It is not necessary to build the Taj Mahal in your backyard: keep it small and effective.

understanding the specific goals of an individual or patient. Whether that person is physically handicapped, seeking mental stimulation, or simply trying to connect with the natural environment on a daily basis, building a garden design that is therapeutic must begin with understanding an individual's specific physical and emotional needs.

Designing a therapeutic garden is usually a collaborative effort. Bring your family and neighbors together and define what it is you want from the garden. Make a list of the three top items that are most important to you based on your health concerns, then incorporate that simplified list into the final design.

Tyson suggests that once the basic goals are understood, then it is possible to prioritize design features such as fountains, pathway needs, and types of plants to be used in the garden. All healing gardens should be organic in nature and have non-toxic plants so that all guests can feel safe and be encouraged to touch anything.

For backyard or side gardens, unify the areas by including hardscaping—paths, patios, and seating areas, for example—that your planting beds will surround. Once you have determined your hardscape and bed design, then consider plants that add texture, shape, variety, color, aroma—anything that adds therapeutic value.

OPPOSITE: This garden view shows an easily traversable walking area that leads to a secret garden. Stimulating curiosity, such as a view of a secret garden at the end of a path, can often encourage efforts in walking or movement. *Photo taken at Chicago Botanic Garden.*

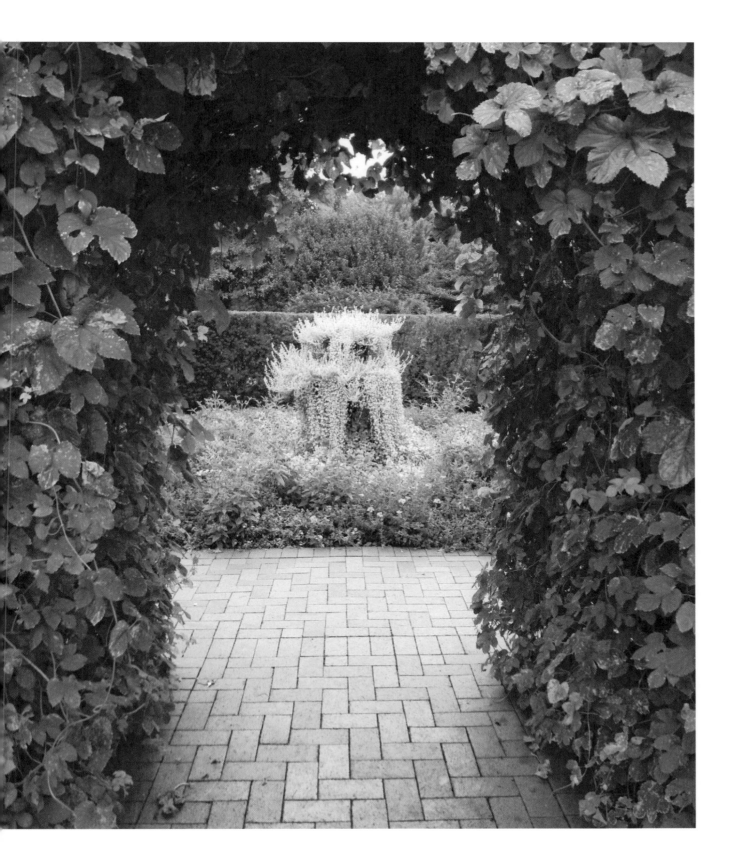

HEALTH ISSUES AND GARDEN SOLUTIONS

As you design, first ask the question, "How do I want the garden to make the patient, visitor, or gardener feel based on their physical and emotional needs?" Less depressed? More emotionally centered? Physically fit? Immersed in beauty? Less chronic pain symptomatic? Nutritionally sound? Connected to nature? Less lonely? The following are a few common considerations.

Wheelchair and Walker Accessibility

If you or a frequent garden visitor has a wheelchair or walker, the most important part of the garden becomes traversing it. Build paths that are smooth, level, firm, and offer a width of at least 5 feet to accommodate a wheelchair's turning ratio. Steep paths make it difficult to traverse as well, so keep paths level.

Increasing Walking Goals

What if you want help to increase your outdoor walking time and distance? Daniel Winterbottom and Amy Wagenfeld suggest in their book *Therapeutic Gardens: Design for Healing Spaces* that marking distances around the garden can increase motivation for the walker. "For those who want to track distance walked, integrate subtle distance markers at strategic points along the paths. Making pathways measured walking trails enables users to partake of outdoor exercise in a controlled environment."

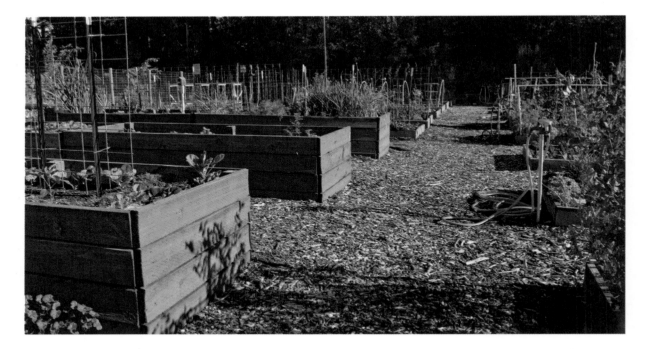

These wide aisles at the Willamette Community Garden in Albany, Oregon, show that it is possible to have a level surface for wheelchair or walker access even with mulch. Keep safety in mind when considering who might be visiting your therapeutic garden.

CHAPTER 12

Building a walking path around your property or neighborhood can be beneficial for you, certainly, but also for the entire neighborhood.

An Arthritis Garden

Whether a gardener has osteoarthritis or rheumatoid arthritis, the need to reduce chronic pain and gain more time doing green activities is critical. A garden designed with these conditions in mind might include elevated vegetable beds and living wall gardens, with drip systems installed so that gardeners do not have to bend in order to plant and water. Easy access to a raised potting area, a level walking path, plus the addition of regular seating throughout the garden to provide rest zones can also help.

Nutritional Concerns

Perhaps your goal is to better your nutritional intake. Build a series of living walls or beds around a small patio, then plant the beds up with ornamental vegetables and herbs in a fashion that encourages participation from your family. Easy access to tools can encourage easy maintenance. Planting a living wall as your kitchen vegetable garden also saves space.

Enabling Garden for Sensory Issues

Building a garden for deaf, blind, or sensory-challenged people might mean installing a space

Perhaps a person who lives with you has poor eyesight. Bringing the plants up to eye level can make a significant difference in their garden viewing experience. This succulent gutter garden is inexpensive and water-smart. Planting on a wall is the perfect way bring a garden up close.

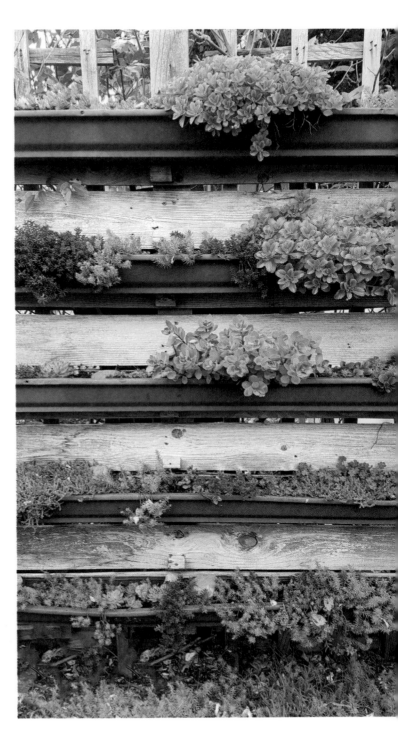

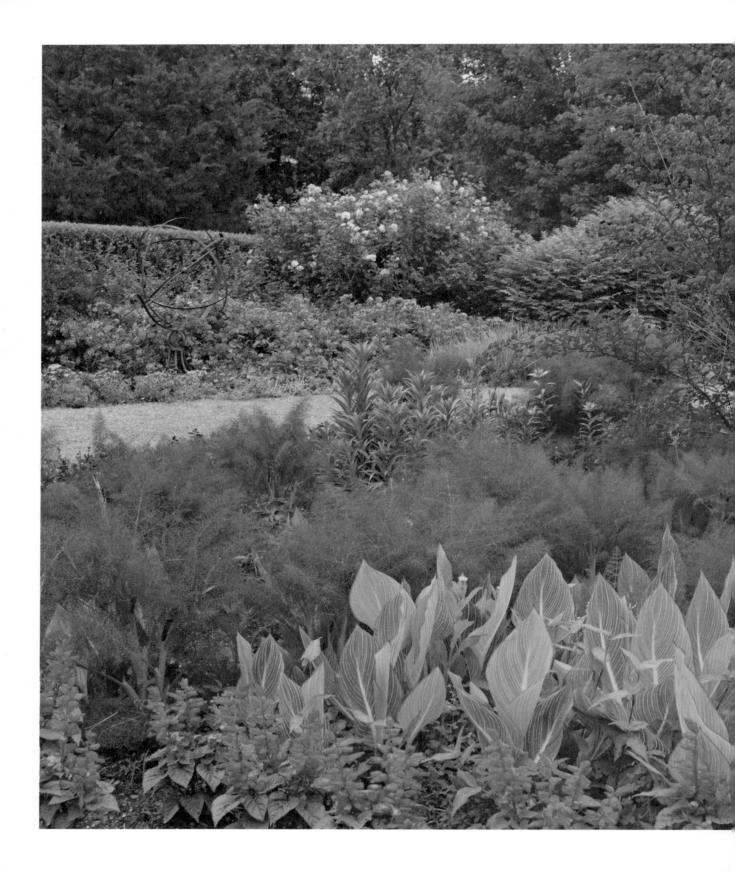

that can enhance the exposure of the five senses. For example, installing a water feature such as a small fountain can enhance the sensory experience. Martha M. Tyson, author of the therapeutic garden design book *The Healing Landscape: Therapeutic Outdoor Environments*, says, "The introduction of water can provide places for birds to gather as well as bring an element of soothing sound to the garden." Additionally, add deliciously fragrant plantings, edible plants, touchable plants with various textures, and colorful foliage can stimulate all the senses. Many sensory gardens also have adult-sized swings.

Garden for the Color Blind

There are different types of color blindness. Many who have this condition have difficulty seeing colors in the red, orange, or purple ranges, for example. This means that their garden experience is unequivocally not what a person with a normal eye would see. For these people, plant lots of white and black plants, which offer contrast. Additionally, based on the specific type of color blindness a person has, incorporate more of the colors they *can* see.

Comfort Garden

For solace, solitude, and sound, a beautiful therapeutic garden can be a seating area that is surrounded by natural sounds and drought-tolerant plantings. Build a native plant garden filled with grasses that move with the wind and require minimal care. When you sit in the area, you will hear the grasses rustling in the breeze. Add wind chimes in tree branches for a bit of music. This type of garden is remarkably low maintenance and can bring immense comfort.

Energizing Exercise Garden

Stimulating exercise gardens often have lots of creative sculptural shapes, either provided by plants or by actual sculpture or colorful art where the eye can rest. Build a garden filled with whimsy and fun, lots of places to sit, and easy access to exercise paths to encourage exercise and group activities. This type of garden can have balance bars or other apparatus installed as well as a large open area for tai chi or yoga.

OPPOSITE: When appropriate for the garden guest, it is very stimulating to create a bold and textural planting combination. This garden design is from P. Allen Smith's Moss Mountain Farm near Little Rock, Arkansas, a delightful place filled with expressive and stimulating gardens designed to energize visitors.

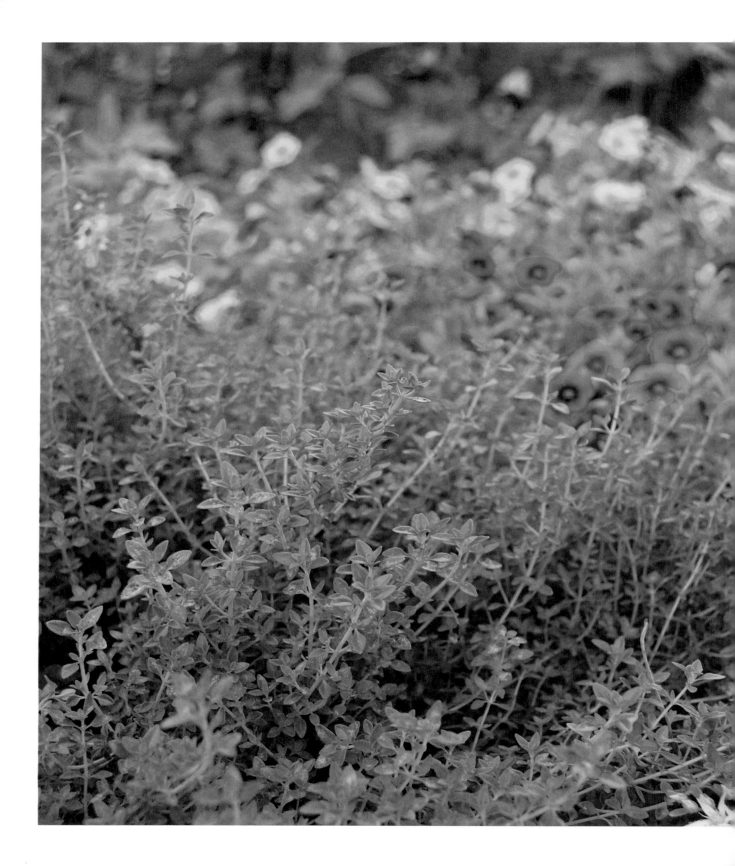

13

FRAGRANCE GARDENING

DANIEL WINTERBOTTOM AND Amy Wagenfeld say in their book, *Therapeutic Gardens: Design for Healing Spaces*, "Highly aromatic herbs are welcome additions to sensory gardens and therapeutic programming at behavioral health and memory care facilities. Beyond the immediate sensory experience, users benefit if plants trigger a sense of wonder because they are unfamiliar or, conversely, a sense of belonging or connection because they are familiar. The Garden of Fragrance in the San Francisco Botanical Garden, designed in 1965 for visitors with visual impairments, has a loop path with 12 stations at beds raised to place a profusion of herbs within reach of wheelchair users. Visitors touch the cascading branches of rosemary leaves on a rock wall, release its scent, and may think of home cooking."

OPPOSITE: One of the most fabulous ways to fragrance garden is to incorporate edible herbs into your containers and ground gardens. Their scent, like this lemon thyme, is mesmerizing and inspires positive thought. Best yet, an herb's flavor is a glorious contribution to your dinner table.

Taking an evening walk through a fragrance garden after a stressful day can completely revive a tired soul. Why not build a scented pathway garden to help you cope with daily stresses?

LIGHTLY SCENTED VERSUS HEAVILY SCENTED GARDENS

Primarily, there are two types of scent gardens: lightly scented and heavily scented. Lightly scented gardens can better support people

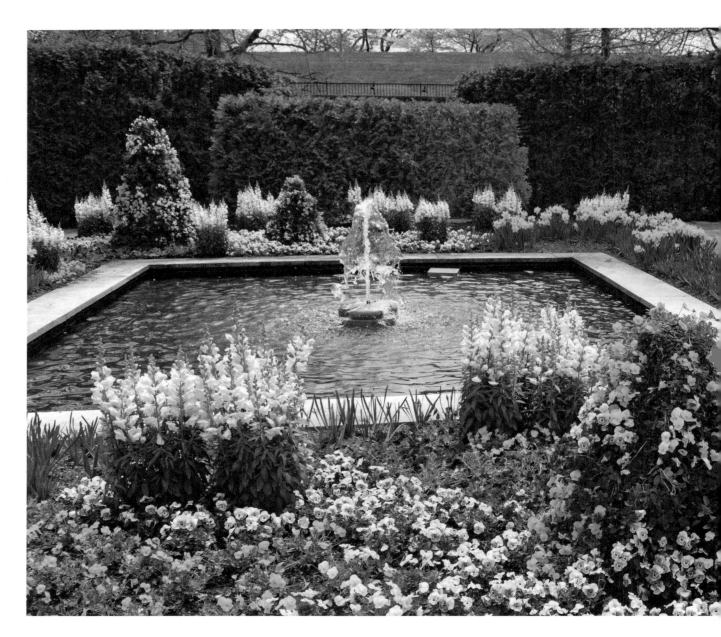

who have sensitivity to strong smells due to cancer treatments, sinus problems, or severe allergies. When going through chemotherapy, for example, many patients have an altered sense of smell and cannot tolerate highly aromatic plants.

In particular, children who are going through chemotherapy can have scent- and tactile-challenges with plants such as lavender. Usually, lavender is known as a healing or calming plant, yet it can be a tad prickly to touch and the scent is very strong. Consider planting lavender well away

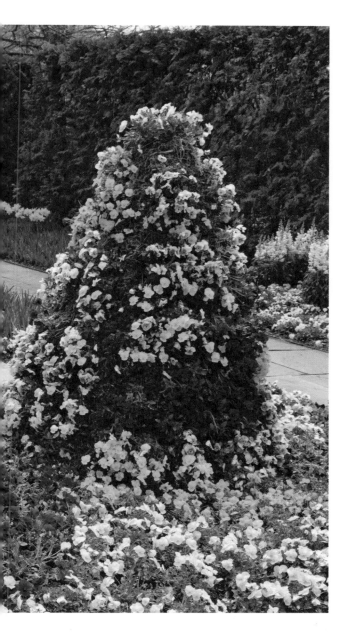

Surrounding yourself with scent can be positive or negative depending on your therapeutic needs. Cancer patients or people with severe allergies, for example, often have sensitivity to strong scents. Therefore, keep your garden guest in mind and perhaps plant a lightly scented garden instead. *Photo taken at Longwood Gardens in Kennett Square, PA.*

Lightly Scented to Odorless Plant List

- Amaryllis
- Anemones
- Begonia
- Calla lilies
- Chocolate cosmos
- Clematis
- Coleus
- Daffodil
- Dahlia
- Daylily
- Dianthus
- Hibiscus
- Hosta
- Hydrangea
- Impatiens
- Knockout Rose 'Sunny'
- Lamb's ears
- Lavender
- Leafy vegetables
- Mullein
- Pansy
- Parsley
- Periwinkle
- Poppy
- Ranunculus
- Strawberry
- Sunflowers
- Violet
- Zinnia

from the primary walking path so that the scent is removed a few steps and the child will not get scratched on their sensitive skin nor overwhelmed with the smell.

For many years in my own garden, I had to avoid heavily scented areas because of severe allergies. My family calls my nose the "super sniffer" because I was remarkably sensitive to smells of any kind, particularly when the smells were chemical in nature. With the changes in my diet, my allergies have become less severe, permitting me to better tolerate strongly scented plants.

The book *Therapeutic Gardens: Design for Healing Spaces* suggests using scent as a brain stimulator when designing therapeutic gardens. "Plants that trigger positive memories or home because of their sweet or savory or unusual scents are especially meaningful to people displaced because of illness, homelessness, or unfamiliar relocation. The evocative scents of sage or rose can engender a comfortable sense of belonging to people in elder care facilities. Used as a team, the smell and very fine texture of chamomile is universally well loved; the fragrance of both it and lavender are found to improve mood and ease stress."

THE NEED FOR POWERFUL SCENTS

Another reason to consider more heavily aromatic plants in your garden is as a benefit to elderly visitors to the garden. The elderly suffer from many sensory changes including a declining ability to smell. This decline triggers taste changes for foods as well, which can make fresh herbs and stronger flavors an important ingredient in kitchen gardening. Heavily aromatic plants can be moved to front and center positions within the garden in order to stimulate a therapeutic reaction among the elderly.

Along with more aromatic fragrances, keep in mind that a scent garden naturally draws people in and encourages them to sit and smell the gorgeous aromas. So, include plenty of stable seating; avoid gliders or rocking chairs if visitors may have balance issues.

Children especially like strong olfactory stimulants, particularly malodorous plants that actually stink, like the corpse flower or western skunk cabbage. However, planting your garden full of plants that smell like death might not encourage happy neighbors. In addition, over-competition among aromas within the garden can be overwhelming and cause attention fatigue. Instead, keep strong-smelling plants separated so each can be enjoyed on its own.

Heavily Scented and Aromatic Plant List

- Angel's trumpet
- Basil
- Crabapple tree
- Four o'clock
- Gardenia
- Heliotrope
- Hyacinth
- Iris
- Jasmine
- Joe-pye weed
- Lavender
- Lemon verbena
- Lilac
- Lily of the valley
- Magnolia tree
- Marigold
- Mint
- Moonflower
- Nicotiana
- Oregano
- Oriental lily
- Peony
- Petunia
- Phlox
- Rosemary
- Roses
- Sage
- Sage 'Scarlet Pineapple'
- Scented geraniums
- Sweet alyssum
- Sweet autumn clematis
- Sweet pea
- Tomatoes
- Tuberose
- Thyme
- White valerian
- Wisteria

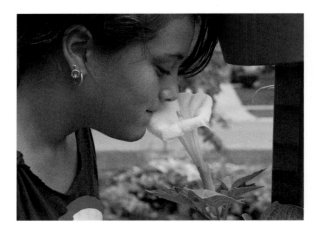

Children, in particular, love strong-smelling plants and flowers. As long as their medical professionals give the go-ahead, consider planting exciting scents to stimulate more contact with plants and the outdoors.

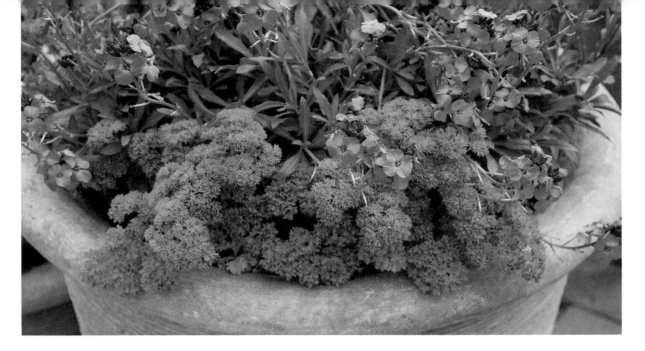

CHAPTER 13

Mixing flowers and herbs together can be delightful to the senses and also supply your kitchen garden. Consider growing herbs such as parsley and basil with your traditional annuals in small therapeutic container gardens.

THE CURE FOR WHAT AILS YOU

Fragrance can be a cure for what ails you. For instance, many people need stress reduction. In this case, planting herbs around a seating area in your garden can strongly enhance your outdoor experience. If, for example, you surround a park bench with rosemary, the scent appears to stimulate a positive energetic reaction. According to a study done by biochemists at the University of Northumbria, a natural compound found in rosemary is absorbed through the nose and into a person's blood plasma. Doctors believe this triggers increased cognitive performances. Imagine a glorious hour spent surrounded by rosemary as you work on your latest computer project. In theory, your computer time could be enhanced dramatically simply by sitting outside where you can find an energetic brain boost with plants.

Lavender has a recognizable scent that the plant exudes from flowers, leaves, and stems. According to the University of Maryland Medical Center, "Scientific evidence suggests that aromatherapy with lavender may slow the activity of the nervous system, improve sleep quality, promote relaxation, and lift mood in people suffering from sleep disorders."

There have been few scientific studies to test the true health values of all herbs. Many agree that scent can either be calming or stimulating based on your own personal reactions and memories related to plant scents. Existing evidentiary studies have had mixed results but seem to point to concentrated mint scents as being a stimulant that improves attention and focus.

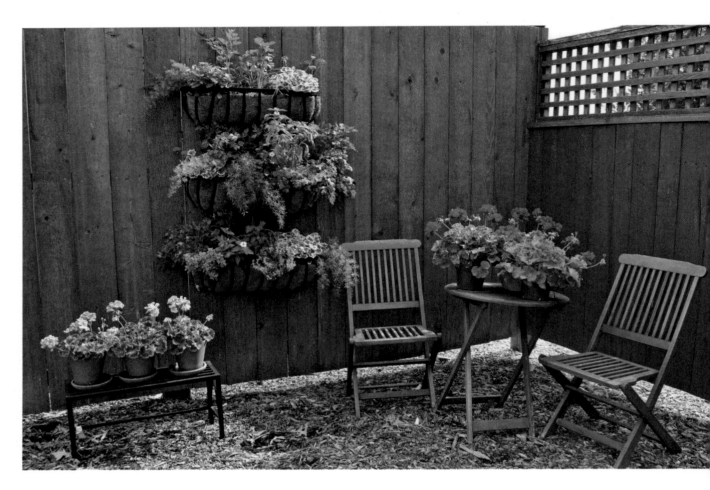

Try growing a scent-themed living wall. This Italian garden has a mix of flowers and specific Italian herbs—parsley, basil, oregano, rosemary, and geraniums.

In a recent scientific study, "Peppermint and Lavender Essential Oils: Are They Therapeutic Aromas for Attention and Memory?" published in *The Internet Journal of Alternative Medicine*, the authors conclusions are clear: "Aroma has direct and indirect psychological effects and the sense of smell stimulates our memory, feelings of creativity, as well as emotions. Peppermint helps in increasing the attention span but memory was not significantly affected. As [whether or not] lavender scent [has a] sedative effect, it decreased the participants' working memory and ability to concentrate."

Therefore, planting containers of mint on your balcony can help increase attention span, and reading near a heavily aromatic garden area filled with mint or rosemary scents might help you to focus. On the other hand, a stressful day might lead you to the lavender beds for a quiet moment of relaxation.

GARDEN FRAGRANCE THEME IDEAS

A lovely way to incorporate scents you like in your fragrance garden is to build a theme when planting. Whether you are in-ground planting, living wall gardening, elevated bed growing, or container gardening, you can try all types of different scented plants.

Many scent gardens are also kitchen-related, so be sure to take advantage of the herbs, vegetables, and edible flowers.

Chili Bowl Garden Ancho chili, cilantro, Mexican oregano, garlic, tomatoes, marigold, Four o'clocks, and petunias.

Caribbean Beach Party Garden Hibiscus, zinnia, cinnamon-scented geranium, clove-scented geranium, garlic, ginger, and allspice.

Tea Party Garden Yarrow, hyssop, lemon verbena, calendula, German chamomile, pineapple sage, betony, stevia, thyme, lavender, peony, lilac, violet, and sweet alyssum.

French Herbs de Provence Garden Rosemary, marjoram, thyme, oregano, sage, tarragon, lavender, savory, sweet pea, sunflowers, and roses.

Herbal Bath and Spa Garden Lavender, mints, sages, chamomile, thymes, parsley, basil, rosemary, roses, strawberry leaves, bay, lemon verbena, and roses.

Italian Garden Italian parsley, basil, oregano, rosemary, tomatoes, green peppers, roses, lemon-scented geranium, and regular geraniums.

Mediterranean Garden Oregano, rosemary, thyme, citrus-scented geranium, coriander, basil, ginger, lavender, jasmine, lamb's ear, garlic, and sage.

The Night Moon Garden Nicotiana, basil, night-blooming jasmine, moonflower, angel's trumpet, and magnolia.

Neapolitan Ice Cream Garden Joe-pye weed, heliotrope, white valerian, sweet autumn clematis, chocolate cosmos, mint-chocolate-scented geranium, pansies, and strawberries.

Rose, Rose, and More Rose Garden Tuberose, lamb's ears, shrub roses, and rose-scented geranium.

Thai Garden Thai basil, Thai pepper, marigolds, mint, lemongrass, cilantro, garlic, curry plant, and Oriental lily.

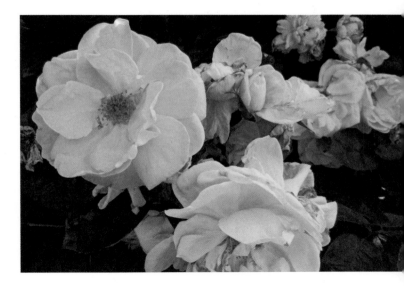

Roses are particularly wonderful memory stimulators. Many people remember the particular scent of their grandmother's roses from when they were a child, for instance, so you can use that memory stimulation as a therapeutic tool. Be sure to research the specific variety of rose you would like to plant because different varieties have different scents.

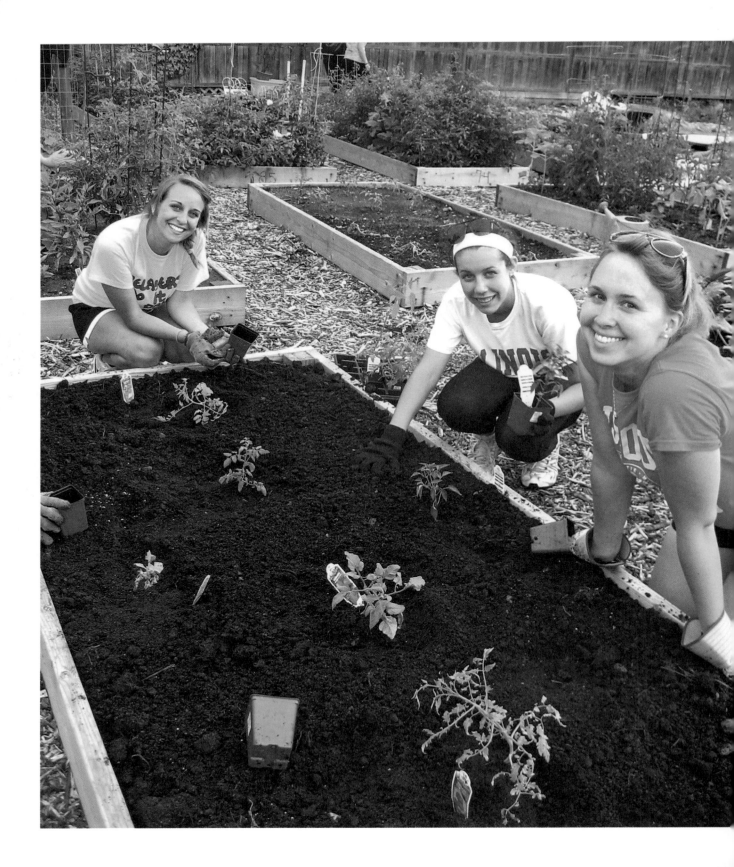

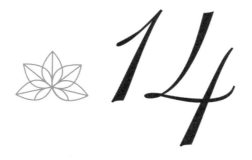

WELLNESS GARDENS AS A SOCIALIZATION TOOL

WELLNESS OR THERAPEUTIC gardens can become a socialization tool to help people—either yourself or people within your community—to reduce social isolation. In our modern society, it is not uncommon for people to be isolated for different reasons. Social isolation is not just about being lonely, but is a deeper and soul-wrenching experience when it means a complete lack of contact with other humans.

OPPOSITE: Social isolation is a major concern in the United States, but community gardens like the Peterson Garden Project are truly making a difference for their neighborhoods by bringing people together to plant and grow.
Peterson Garden Project (PetersonGarden.org).

SOCIAL ISOLATION

In the journal *Perspectives on Psychological Science*, a study ("Loneliness and Social Isolation as Risk Factors for Mortality," March 2015) showed that the feeling of loneliness can intensify the risk of dying by 26 percent compared to those who are not lonely. However, complete social isolation was found to be far more detrimental, increasing mortality risk up to 32 percent.

In the United States, more people are living alone than ever before. With social media and cell phone texting at an all-time high, we tend to use digital means to avoid committing to the more

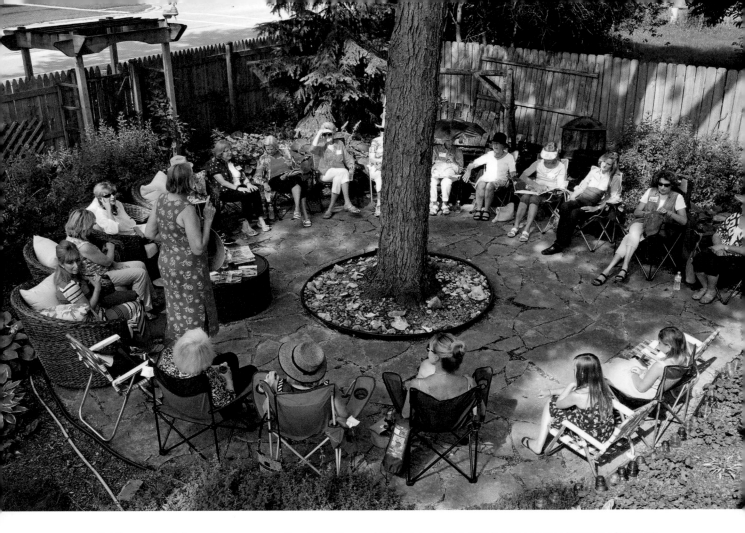

Holding garden club meetings or community get-togethers outside in your home garden is a great way to bring people in your neighborhood out of their homes and into your circle.

time-consuming relationships that encourage us to meet face to face. In recent history, GlobalWorkplaceAnalytics.com reports that approximately 3.7 million US employees have started telecommuting or working from home, some part-time and many full-time, which further isolates people from direct human contact.

When discussion first began about social isolation in the modern world, it was assumed that the elderly or medical shut-ins made up the vast majority of isolated individuals. Yet Duke University and the University of Arizona researchers discovered after interviewing a sampling of 1,500 people of all different ages that more than 50 percent of them said they had no one to talk to in order to share their successes or personal troubles.

Veterans, in particular, can be at risk for social isolation because they often have fragmented

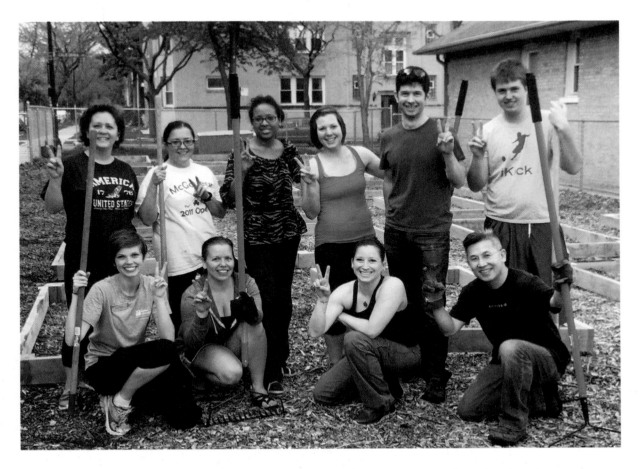

Isolation and depression can lead to extreme loneliness. Building and maintaining a garden together, either at your home or through a community garden like the Peterson Garden Project in Chicago, Illinois, can truly make a difference for someone who is isolated. Connecting with other people can help them be less lonely and feel as if they are included in a caring environment.
Peterson Garden Project (PetersonGarden.org).

medical care, disabling physical injuries, and psychological trauma from their experiences in the military. Isolation can happen because of self-blame, drug addiction, and many other reasons as well. In the end, when we live in social isolation we begin to feel overwhelmingly hopeless and as if others do not care about us.

Twelve million people over the age of 65 are living alone, and a large percentage of those older adults are women. Social isolation is linked to depression, impaired mobility, arthritis, and poor cognitive performance and decline. This frequently means that seniors who are isolated are more likely to need long-term home care or

WELLNESS GARDENS AS A SOCIALIZATION TOOL

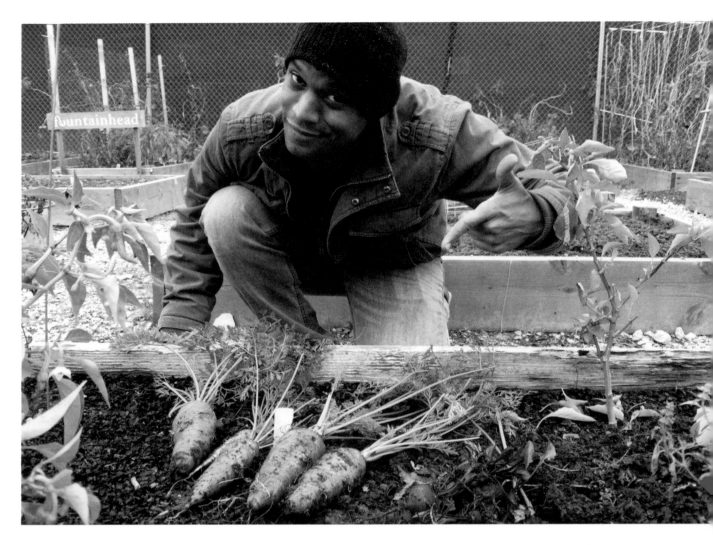

Community gardens do more than simply bring people together to socialize. They provide a place where the community can exercise and grow healthy food. This builds a sense of pride and ownership that can benefit an entire area. *Peterson Garden Project (PetersonGarden.org).*

to enter nursing homes. Because social isolation continues to be a large and striking problem amongst the elderly, building social contacts and staying active after retirement is particularly important. Gardening and horticultural therapy can help.

THE CURE FOR LONELINESS

Loneliness in itself is a deeply personal existence. Some loneliness, depression, and isolation issues cannot be tackled without a health professional, counselor, or caregiver to intervene. However, in many cases, combatting loneliness is as simple as connecting with an isolated or depressed neighbor or friend and inviting them to share time with you.

If the person you are concerned about is not sure what they might like to do to reduce their isolation, start by asking him what his interests are. Suggest you do an activity together that speaks to his interests and likes. Share herbs or vegetables from your garden to kick off the conversation. If gardening is not an interest, ask if he might come and sit in the sunlight with you to chat while you weed or work soil. Often people have a difficult time getting out of the habit of isolating themselves and need a helping hand to find new ways to explore the world.

Sharing time together, working on green activities such as gardening projects or a community garden, walking in nature and garden-like locations, and environmental conservation work are intimate parts of a wellness lifestyle. In fighting isolation, the activities are a two-fer: they function as a social connector so you can talk and spend time with another human being and as an anti-depressant because spending time outside in nature and sunlight functions is a mood elevator.

FINDING YOUR WELLNESS

Whether you are working in an office, living life at your home, or helping your community, it is possible to live a wellness lifestyle. Gardening is a great step toward that wellness. You can grow healthy herbs and vegetables. You can exercise or walk regularly out of doors. Unmistakably, the real secret to finding your wellness is committing your heart and soul to eating more nutritiously with an eye to your personal health issues and to find that outdoor place where you can connect with nature therapeutically via green activities.

This amazing experience of combining diet, walking, and gardening has changed my life and my future. I have discovered a lifestyle with significantly less pain where every day feels a little better, and I enjoy and appreciate my daily existence more than I ever did in the past. I hope this book, *The Wellness Garden*, will inspire you to take the first steps toward healthier living that features regular exercise and a mindful, anti-inflammatory diet.

What is wellness? It is living a mindful life filled with good nutrition and regular exercise in the open air. Wellness embraces an ever-changing and expanding lifestyle that involves eating healthier, exercising regularly, and establishing an emotional balance in life.

While many think wellness is a destination, I say it is a journey where every moment is inhaled and exhaled to create the rhythm of our lives. Find your wellness journey every day of your life.

You can do this.

I believe in you.

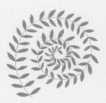

DEDICATION AND ACKNOWLEDGMENTS

**I dedicate this book to Kelsey and Sam.
They have inspired me to have a lifestyle where I live well,
love wholly, and laugh often.**

Special thanks go to my dear husband and family: I love you with all my heart!

Cool Springs Press has the best and most wonderful team ever—Mark Johanson, my editor, is also a treasured friend. I am eternally grateful to you, Mark. Your support is needed and appreciated. My marketing team, Steve Roth and Lola Honeybone, are terrific. My team includes Cathy Lane and Alyssa Bluhm—thank you so very much for guiding me. I am especially grateful for the artists, designers, and assistants who help me put these books together with their colossal talent.

I thank Rick Bayless and Ron Finley for allowing me to feature their unique and powerful stories in this book. Thanks to Niki Jabbour for enabling me to get more insight into winter vegetable growing and harvesting.

Part of compiling a book is spending many long and lonely hours shooting photos at hundreds of locations. *The Wellness Garden* has photos of many plants or locations from Ball Horticultural, Biltmore Estate, Chanticleer, Costa Farms, Moss Mountain Farm, Peterson Garden Project, The Planter's Palette garden center, WoollyPocket. com, and so many other locations and community gardens—thank you one and all.

Special thanks to Diana Stoll, Jenny Nybro Peterson, Terri Curtis, Jacque Gregory, Laura Eubanks, Lamanda Joy, Liz Donaghy, Jane Schwartz Gates, David Sylvian-Czajkowski, Diane Blazek, Kylee Baumle, Christina Salwitz, and Helen Weis for helping me with photos and life in general. I am grateful to you all for your kind friendship and guidance. And to Bruce Baker and Bob Denman for teaching me so much about the ergonomics of tools.

Enormous and loving thanks to Deepa Deshmukh, my nutritionist and dear friend. She opened my eyes and taught me that food is medicine. I am now living with significantly less pain and a happier existence because of her inspiration. Deepa is generous to a fault and has kindly shared her team of researchers who helped me discover the detailed nutritive value of beans and vegetables—thank you to Anam Fatima, Humna Usmani, and Nicole Michehl.

Most especially I want to thank all my wonderful followers who come to my speeches, who order my books, and who are in touch with me via social media every single day. Your support made it possible for me to keep going when my health was at the darkest point. I'm thrilled you stuck with me and cheered me on. I love you!

If I can discover less pain, more health, and a wellness lifestyle, I know that you can too. I am grateful for you and I believe in you. Keep moving forward—do not give up!

INDEX

CONVERSIONS

Converting Measurements

To Convert:	To:	Multiply by:
Inches	Millimeters	25.4
Inches	Centimeters	2.54
Feet	Meters	0.305
Yards	Meters	0.914
Miles	Kilometers	1.609
Square inches	Square centimeters	6.45
Square feet	Square meters	0.093
Square yards	Square meters	0.836
Cubic inches	Cubic centimeters	16.4
Cubic feet	Cubic meters	0.0283
Cubic yards	Cubic meters	0.765
Pints (US)	Liters	0.473 (Imp. 0.568)
Quarts (US)	Liters	0.946 (Imp. 1.136)
Gallons (US)	Liters	3.785 (Imp. 4.546)
Ounces	Grams	28.4
Pounds	Kilograms	0.454
Tons	Metric tons	0.907

To Convert:	To:	Multiply by:
Millimeters	Inches	0.039
Centimeters	Inches	0.394
Meters	Feet	3.28
Meters	Yards	1.09
Kilometers	Miles	0.621
Square centimeters	Square inches	0.155
Square meters	Square feet	10.8
Square meters	Square yards	1.2
Cubic centimeters	Cubic inches	0.061
Cubic meters	Cubic feet	35.3
Cubic meters	Cubic yards	1.31
Liters	Pints (US)	2.114 (Imp. 1.76)
Liters	Quarts (US)	1.057 (Imp. 0.88)
Liters	Gallons (US)	0.264 (Imp. 0.22)
Grams	Ounces	0.035
Kilograms	Pounds	2.2
Metric tons	Tons	1.1

Converting Temperatures

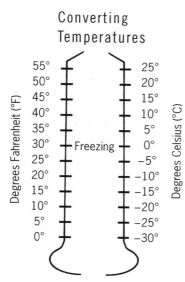

Degrees Fahrenheit (°F): 55° 50° 45° 40° 35° 30° (Freezing) 25° 20° 15° 10° 5° 0°

Degrees Celsius (°C): 25° 20° 15° 10° 5° 0° (Freezing) −5° −10° −15° −20° −25° −30°

Metric Equivalent

Inches (in.)	1/64	1/32	1/25	1/16	1/8	1/4	3/8	2/5	1/2	5/8	3/4	7/8	1
Feet (ft.)													
Yards (yd.)													
Millimeters (mm)	0.40	0.79	1	1.59	3.18	6.35	9.53	10	12.7	15.9	19.1	22.2	25.4
Centimeters (cm)								0.95	1	1.27	1.59	1.91	2.22	2.54
Meters (m)													

Inches (in.)	2	3	4	5	6	7	8	9	10	11	12	36	39.4
Feet (ft.)											1	3	3½
Yards (yd.)												1	1½
Millimeters (mm)	50.8	76.2	101.6	127	152	178	203	229	254	279	305	914	1,000
Centimeters (cm)	5.08	7.62	10.16	12.7	15.2	17.8	20.3	22.9	25.4	27.9	30.5	91.4	100
Meters (m)											.30	.91	1.00

°F to°C: Subtract 32 from the Fahrenheit temperature reading. Then mulitply that number by 5/9.
For example, 77°F − 32 = 45. 45 × 5/9 = 25°C.
°C to°F: Multiply the Celsius temperature reading by 9/5, then add 32.
For example, 25°C × 9/5 = 45. 45 + 32 = 77°F.

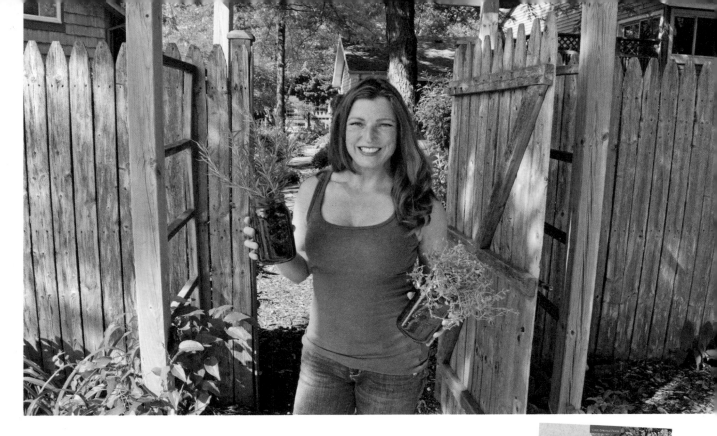

MEET SHAWNA CORONADO

Shawna Coronado is a wellness and green-living lifestyle advocate. As an author, photographer, influencer, and media host, Shawna campaigns globally for social good and health awareness. With a "make a difference" focus on sustainable home living, organic gardening, and healthy food recipes built to inspire, Shawna hopes to stimulate positive changes for her community and the world.

Her garden and eco-adventures have been featured in many media venues including radio and television. Shawna's successful organic-living photographs and stories have been shared on and off in many international home and garden magazines and in multiple books. You can meet Shawna by connecting online with her on her blog and website at www.shawnacoronado.com.

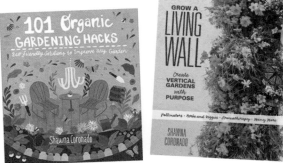

WANT TO READ MORE of Shawna Coronado's organic, green, and ground-breaking books on wellness and smart sustainable growing?

Find *101 Organic Garden Hacks: Eco-Friendly Solutions to Improve Any Garden* and *Grow a Living Wall: Create Vertical Gardens with Purpose* online and at bookstores everywhere.